Minor Injury and Minor Illness at a Glance

Edited by

Francis Morris

Consultant in Emergency Medicine
Sheffield Teaching Hospitals
NHS Foundation Trust
Sheffield

Jim Wardrope

Consultant in Emergency Medicine
Sheffield Teaching Hospitals
NHS Foundation Trust
Sheffield

and

Shammi Ramlakhan

Consultant in Adult and Paediatric Emergency Medicine
Sheffield Children's Hospital;
Sheffield Teaching Hospitals
NHS Foundation Trust
Sheffiled

WILEY Blackwell

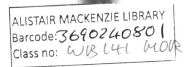
Library of Congress Cataloging-in-Publication Data

Minor injury and minor illness at a glance / edited by Francis Morris, Jim Wardrope, and Shammi Ramlakhan.
      p. ; cm. – (At a glance series)
  Includes bibliographical references and index.
  ISBN 978-1-118-26135-4 (pbk.)
  I. Morris, Francis, editor.   II. Wardrope, Jim, editor.   III. Ramlakhan, Shammi, editor.
IV. Series: At a glance series (Oxford, England)
  [DNLM: 1. Diagnosis.   2. Wounds and Injuries–diagnosis. WB 141]
  RD93
  617.1–dc23
                                    2014000048

A catalogue record for this book is available from the British Library.

Wiley also publishes its books in a variety of electronic formats. Some content that appears in print may not be available in electronic books.

Cover image: © bojan fatur (iStock photo ID: 15530769)
Cover design by Wiley

Set in 9/11.5 pt Times by Toppan Best-set Premedia Limited
Printed and bound in Malaysia by Vivar Printing Sdn Bhd

1   2014

Contents

Preface

This book is aimed the assessment and treatment of 'minor' conditions. However, patients may present with apparently minor symptoms that actually are the early signs of a more serious problem. A systematic approach gives you the best chance of reaching an accurate diagnosis. There is often pressure to work fast, and thus it is even more important to adopt a slick and efficient structure to assessment.

Each chapter deals with a body or system area. The general approach to the patient is described and then some detail given for common conditions. 'Red flags', symptoms or signs that might indicate a serious condition, are highlighted.

The chapters end with 'Diagnoses not to be missed' – pathologies that may masquerade as minor problems but carry real risks of death, disability for the patient and months or years of worry to you if you happen to miss such conditions.

The care of 'minor' conditions may be routine, but it should never be boring.

Francis Morris
Jim Wardrope
Shammi Ramlakhan

Contributors

Helen Cannings
Specialist Registrar Emergency Medicine
Sheffield Teaching Hospitals NHS Foundation Trust
Sheffield

Michael Davey
Emergency Department Clinical Nurse Educator
Sheffield Teaching Hospitals NHS Trust
Sheffield

Nicki Doddridge
Consultant in Acute Medicine
Sheffield Teaching Hospitals NHS Trust
Sheffield

Claire L Fitzpatrick
Consultant in Emergency Medicine
Glasgow Royal Infirmary
Glasgow

Chris Fitzsimmons
Consultant in Paediatric Emergency Medicine
Sheffield Children's Hospital
Sheffield

Alan Fletcher
Consultant in Emergency Medicine and Acute Medicine
Sheffield Teaching Hospitals NHS Foundation Trust
Sheffield

Clare Ginnis
Senior Trainee in Paediatric Emergency Medicine
South Yorkshire and Humber Deanery

Mohamed Gossiel
Consultant in Emergency Medicine
Sheffield Teaching Hospitals NHS Foundation Trust
Sheffield

Richard Griffiths
Specialist Registrar
Barnsley Hospital NHS Foundation Trust
Barnsley

Abu Hassan
Consultant in Emergency Medicine
Northern General Hospital
Sheffield Teaching Hospitals NHS Foundation Trust
Sheffield

Sherif Hemaya
Consultant in Emergency Medicine
Northern General Hospital
Sheffield Teaching Hospitals NHS Foundation Trust
Sheffield

Robert W Jones
Specialist Registrar
Emergency Medicine
Sheffield Teaching Hospitals
Sheffield

Faheem Khan
Consultant, Emergency Medicine and Intensive Care
Royal Wolverhampton Hospital NHS Trust
Wolverhampton

Avril J Kuhrt
Consultant in Emergency Medicine
Northern General Hospital
Sheffield

Andrew McCoye
General Practitioner
Sheffield

Julie Perrin
Nurse Consultant
Emergency Care
Sheffield Teaching Hospitals NHS Foundation Trust
Sheffield

Alicia Ramtahal
General Practitioner
Sheffield

Ian Sammy
Senior Lecturer in Emergency Medicine
The University of the West Indies
St Augustine, Trinidad

Christopher M Smith
Specialist Trainee in Emergency Medicine
Hull and East Yorkshire Hospitals NHS Trust
Hull

Sarah Stabon
Emergency Nurse Practitioner
Sheffield Teaching Hospitals NHS Foundation Trust
Sheffield

Melanie Stevens
Emergency Nurse Practitioner
Sheffield Teaching Hospitals NHS Foundation Trust
Sheffield

Kathryn Whittle
Obstetrics and Gynaecology Registrar
Sheffield Teaching Hospitals NHS Foundation Trust
Sheffield

Penelope Williams
Specialist Registrar in Dermatology
Royal Devon and Exeter NHS Foundation Trust
Exeter

How to use your textbook

Features contained within your textbook
Each topic is presented in a double-page spread with clear, easy-to-follow diagrams supported by succinct explanatory text.

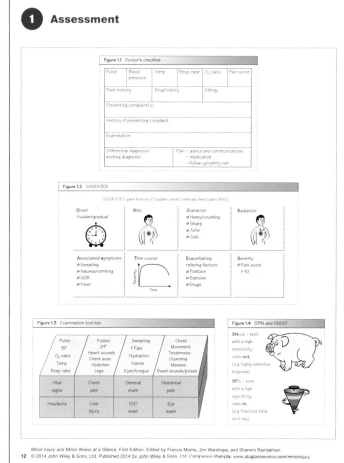

1 Assessment

Objectives
This book is aimed the assessment and treatment of 'minor' conditions. However, patients may present with apparently minor symptoms that are the start of a more serious problem. A systematic approach gives you the best chance of reaching an accurate diagnosis. There is often pressure to work fast; thus, it is even more important to adopt a slick and efficient structure to assessment.

A pilot does not take off before a check of vital systems has been made; the effects of error could be lethal. Equally, you need to have a checklist in your mind before discharging a patient; error could be lethal (see Figure 1.1).

System of assessment
History
• **Presenting complaint(s).** It is self-evident that you need to address the patient's main symptom(s). These should be listed.
• **Symptoms.** Individual symptoms and how to elicit a full history of that symptom are expanded in each chapter. Pain is a very common symptom; thus, a systematic method of obtaining a pain history is summarised in Figure 1.2 (SOCRATES).
• **Past history, drugs, allergy.** The patient may have had similar symptoms before and indeed had treatment (previous diagnoses may not be relevant/correct). Major illness (e.g. diabetes, lung/heart disease) may have a bearing on diagnosis and management. Key medications (e.g. warfarin, cardiac and diabetic drugs) need to be recorded.

Examination
• **Vital signs.** Disturbance of vital signs is one of the most important **red flags**. All early-warning scores to highlight serious illness are based on vital signs. **Vital signs are vital.**
Early-warning scores are now commonly used to identify patients with an increased risk of serious deterioration in their condition. These scores emphasise the importance of abnormal vital signs.
• **General exam.** Learn to recognise the ill patient. The signs are subtle, the patient is pale, dark eyes, dry tongue, looks anxious. *Patients who look ill need careful assessment.*
• **Exam routines.** Develop a number of 'exam routines' for common presentations such as chest pain, injury, headache (Figure 1.3).

Investigations
• **Do you really need a test?** Investigations should only be carried out if they are necessary. Once a patient is assessed and a clinical is diagnosis reached, further investigations may not be necessary (tonsillitis, cellulitis, paronychia).
• **Sensitivity and specificity** (Figure 1.4). Some investigations have a high specificity (if the test is positive then the patient has the disease – e.g. an obvious fracture of the tibia in a patient with a leg injury). However, some tests, such as d-dimer and highly sensitive troponin, are not specific (a patient with a positive d-dimer has a less than 50% chance of having a deep vein thrombosis (DVT)). Routine ordering of tests with poor sensitivity will require a number of patients having to have further expensive or invasive investigations (see Figure 1.3).
• **Clinical decision rules.** These are evidence-based pathways that can help you decide if a patient requires investigation. These will be discussed in detail where appropriate (e.g. Ottawa ankle rules).

Types of investigations
'Quick and easy' investigations that should be within the scope of any minor illness/injury service include electrocardiogram (ECG), urine dipstick, urine pregnancy test and strip testing for blood glucose. Access X-rays are essential in the assessment of all but the most trivial minor injuries.

Computed tomography scans, magnetic resonance imaging, bone scan and ultrasound are mostly hospital-based tests for more complex or serious problems.

Blood tests are not commonly required for minor illness or injury, but exceptions include chest pain and rule out pathways for DVT.

Microbiology, such as urine/throat/wound/sputum specimens, is required to confirm the diagnosis. However, the results will not be immediately available and treatment is often commenced empirically. Follow up of results is essential.

Interpreting results of investigations
Always use the result of a test as part of the picture. The result may be unequivocal, usually when the test is positive and the test has a high specificity (e.g. the obvious fracture on X-ray). More often the result may be less certain and other parts of evidence have to be taken into account.

Pitfalls in the interpretation of investigations include:
• inexperience or lack of skill in interpretation (e.g. missing a fracture on an X-ray);
• placing too much emphasis on an equivocal test (e.g. diagnosing a urinary tract infection in a patient with abdominal pain on the basis of a few leucocytes on strip testing);
• being unaware of the implications of negative tests (a normal ECG does not rule out an myocardial infarction/acute coronary syndrome);
• ignoring the results of a positive test (e.g. saying that a raised d-dimer in a patient with chest pain is due to a chest infection);
• not following up an abnormal result (delay in acting on an abnormal X-ray report).

Differential diagnosis/working diagnosis
In the acute consultation diagnosis may be imprecise and very often no diagnosis is reached.

Adopt a method of considering possible diagnoses for the presenting complaint:
• Have potentially life- or limb-threatening conditions been ruled out? Is there enough clinical evidence to indicate that these have been ruled out or that they are very unlikely?
• What is the most likely diagnosis?
• Do you need more advice, time or investigation to confirm the diagnosis?

Minor Injury and Minor Illness at a Glance, First Edition. Edited by Francis Morris, Jim Wardrope, and Shammi Ramlakhan.

Assessment **System of care** 13

▶ This icon indicates conditions requiring immediate attention.

This icon indicates that you can read more on a topic by visiting the companion website.

The anytime, anywhere textbook
Wiley E-Text

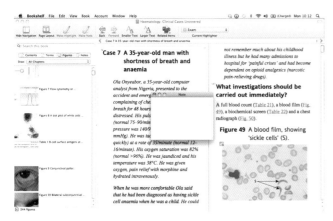

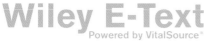

CourseSmart

Your book is also available to purchase as a **Wiley E-Text: Powered by VitalSource** version – a digital, interactive version of this book which you own as soon as you download it.

Your **Wiley E-Text** allows you to:

Search: Save time by finding terms and topics instantly in your book, your notes, even your whole library (once you've downloaded more textbooks)

Note and Highlight: Colour code, highlight and make digital notes right in the text so you can find them quickly and easily

Organize: Keep books, notes and class materials organized in folders inside the application

Share: Exchange notes and highlights with friends, classmates and study groups

Upgrade: Your textbook can be transferred when you need to change or upgrade computers

Link: Link directly from the page of your interactive textbook to all of the material contained on the companion website

The **Wiley E-Text** version will also allow you to copy and paste any photograph or illustration into assignments, presentations and your own notes.

To access your Wiley E-Text:
• Visit **www.vitalsource.com/software/bookshelf/downloads** to download the Bookshelf application to your computer, laptop, tablet or mobile device.
• Open the Bookshelf application on your computer and register for an account.
• Follow the registration process.

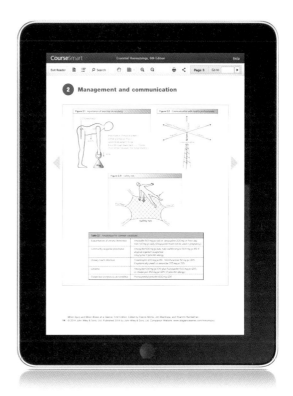

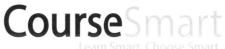

CourseSmart gives you instant access (via computer or mobile device) to this Wiley-Blackwell e-book and its extra electronic functionality, at 40% off the recommended retail print price. See all the benefits at: **www.coursesmart.com/students**

Instructors . . . receive your own digital desk copies!
CourseSmart also offers instructors an immediate, efficient, and environmentally friendly way to review this book for your course.
For more information visit **www.coursesmart.com/instructors**.
With CourseSmart, you can create lecture notes quickly with copy and paste, and share pages and notes with your students. Access your

CourseSmart digital book from your computer or mobile device instantly for evaluation, class preparation, and as a teaching tool in the classroom.
Simply sign in at **http://instructors.coursesmart.com/bookshelf** to download your Bookshelf and get started. To request your desk copy, hit 'Request Online Copy' on your search results or book product page.

We hope you enjoy using your new book. Good luck with your studies!

About the companion website

Don't forget to visit the companion website for this book:

  **www.ataglanceseries.com/minorinjury**

There you will find valuable material designed to enhance your learning, including:
• Interactive short answer questions
• Interactive flashcards with on/off label functionality
• PowerPoint slides of the figures from the book
Scan this QR code to visit the companion website:

Figure 1.1 Doctor's checklist

Pulse	Blood pressure	Temp	Resp. rate	O₂ sats	Pain score
Past history		Drug history		Allergy	
Presenting complaint(s)					
History of presenting complaint					
Examination					
Differential diagnosis/ working diagnosis		Plan – advice and communications – medication – follow-up/safety net			

Figure 1.2 SOCRATES

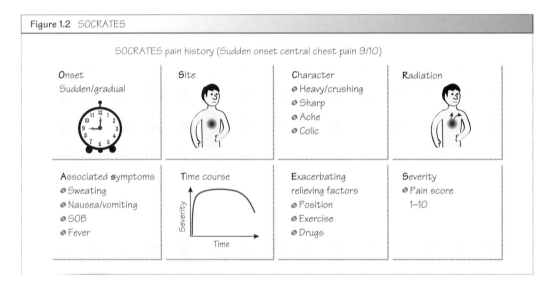

SOCRATES pain history (Sudden onset central chest pain 9/10)

Onset
Sudden/gradual

Site

Character
- Heavy/crushing
- Sharp
- Ache
- Colic

Radiation

Associated symptoms
- Sweating
- Nausea/vomiting
- SOB
- Fever

Time course

Exacerbating relieving factors
- Position
- Exercise
- Drugs

Severity
- Pain score
  1–10

Figure 1.3 Examination tool box

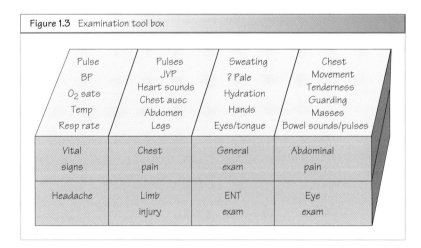

Pulse BP O₂ sats Temp Resp rate	Pulses JVP Heart sounds Chest ausc Abdomen Legs	Sweating ? Pale Hydration Hands Eyes/tongue	Chest Movement Tenderness Guarding Masses Bowel sounds/pulses
Vital signs	Chest pain	General exam	Abdominal pain
Headache	Limb injury	ENT exam	Eye exam

Figure 1.4 SPIN and SNOUT

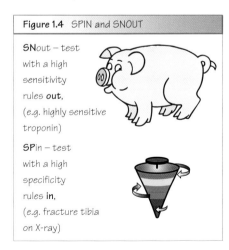

SNout – test with a high sensitivity rules **out**, (e.g. highly sensitive troponin)

SPin – test with a high specificity rules **in**, (e.g. fracture tibia on X-ray)

Minor Injury and Minor Illness at a Glance, First Edition. Edited by Francis Morris, Jim Wardrope, and Shammi Ramlakhan.

Objectives

This book is aimed the assessment and treatment of 'minor' conditions. However, patients may present with apparently minor symptoms that are the start of a more serious problem. A systematic approach gives you the best chance of reaching an accurate diagnosis. There is often pressure to work fast; thus, it is even more important to adopt a slick and efficient structure to assessment.

A pilot does not take off before a check of vital systems has been made; the effects of error could be lethal. Equally, you need to have a checklist in your mind before discharging a patient; error could be lethal (see Figure 1.1).

System of assessment
History
• **Presenting complaint(s).** It is self-evident that you need to address the patient's main symptom(s). These should be listed.
• **Symptoms.** Individual symptoms and how to elicit a full history of that symptom are expanded in each chapter. Pain is a very common symptom; thus, a systematic method of obtaining a pain history is summarised in Figure 1.2 (SOCRATES).
• **Past history, drugs, allergy.** The patient may have had similar symptoms before and indeed had treatment (previous diagnoses may not be relevant/correct). Major illness (e.g. diabetes, lung/heart disease) may have a bearing on diagnosis and management. Key medications (e.g. warfarin, cardiac and diabetic drugs) need to be recorded.

Examination
• **Vital signs.** Disturbance of vital signs is one of the most important **red flags**. All early-warning scores to highlight serious illness are based on vital signs. **Vital signs are vital.**
Early-warning scores are now commonly used to identify patients with an increased risk of serious deterioration in their condition. These scores emphasise the importance of abnormal vital signs.
• **General exam.** Learn to recognise the ill patient. The signs are subtle, the patient is pale, dark eyes, dry tongue, looks anxious. *Patients who look ill need careful assessment.*
• **Exam routines.** Develop a number of 'exam routines' for common presentations such as chest pain, injury, headache (Figure 1.3).

Investigations
• **Do you really need a test?** Investigations should only be carried out if they are necessary. Once a patient is assessed and a clinical is diagnosis reached, further investigations may not be necessary (tonsillitis, cellulitis, paronychia).
• **Sensitivity and specificity** (Figure 1.4). Some investigations have a high specificity (if the test is positive then the patient has the disease – e.g. an obvious fracture of the tibia in a patient with a leg injury). However, some tests, such as d-dimer and highly sensitive troponin, are not specific (a patient with a positive d-dimer has a less than 50% chance of having a deep vein thrombosis (DVT)). Routine ordering of tests with poor sensitivity will require a number of patients having to have further expensive or invasive investigations (see Figure 1.3).
• **Clinical decision rules.** These are evidence-based pathways that can help you decide if a patient requires investigation. These will be discussed in detail where appropriate (e.g. Ottawa ankle rules).

Types of investigations
'Quick and easy' investigations that should be within the scope of any minor illness/injury service include electrocardiogram (ECG), urine dipstick, urine pregnancy test and strip testing for blood glucose. Access X-rays are essential in the assessment of all but the most trivial minor injuries.

Computed tomography scans, magnetic resonance imaging, bone scan and ultrasound are mostly hospital-based tests for more complex or serious problems.

Blood tests are not commonly required for minor illness or injury, but exceptions include chest pain and rule out pathways for DVT.

Microbiology, such as urine/throat/wound/sputum specimens, is required to confirm the diagnosis. However, the results will not be immediately available and treatment is often commenced empirically. Follow up of results is essential.

Interpreting results of investigations
Always use the result of a test as part of the picture. The result may be unequivocal, usually when the test is positive and the test has a high specificity (e.g. the obvious fracture on X-ray). More often the result may be less certain and other parts of evidence have to be taken into account.

Pitfalls in the interpretation of investigations include:
• inexperience or lack of skill in interpretation (e.g. missing a fracture on an X-ray);
• placing too much emphasis on an equivocal test (e.g. diagnosing a urinary tract infection in a patient with abdominal pain on the basis of a few leucocytes on strip testing);
• being unaware the implications of negative tests (a normal ECG does not rule out an myocardial infarction/acute coronary syndrome);
• ignoring the results of a positive test (e.g. saying that a raised d-dimer in a patient with chest pain is due to a chest infection);
• not following up an abnormal result (delay in acting on an abnormal X-ray report).

Differential diagnosis/working diagnosis
In the acute consultation diagnosis may be imprecise and very often no diagnosis is reached.

Adopt a method of considering possible diagnoses for the presenting complaint:
• Have potentially life- or limb-threatening conditions been ruled out? Is there enough clinical evidence to indicate that these have been ruled out or that they are very unlikely?
• What is the most likely diagnosis?
• Do you need more advice, time or investigation to confirm the diagnosis?

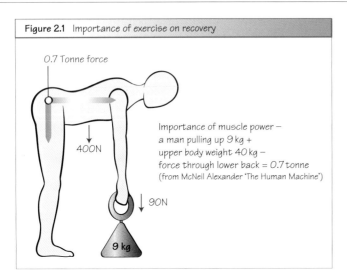

Figure 2.1 Importance of exercise on recovery

0.7 Tonne force

400N

90N

9 kg

Importance of muscle power –
a man pulling up 9 kg +
upper body weight 40 kg –
force through lower back = 0.7 tonne
(from McNeil Alexander 'The Human Machine')

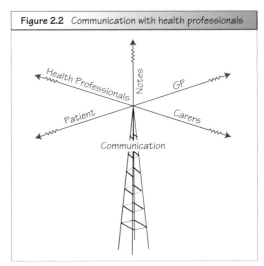

Figure 2.2 Communication with health professionals

Health Professionals

Notes

GP

Patient

Carers

Communication

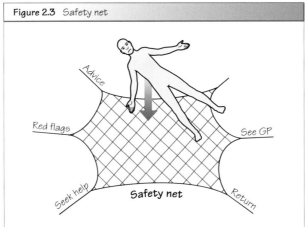

Figure 2.3 Safety net

Advice

Red flags

See GP

Seek help

Return

Safety net

Table 2.1 Antibiotics for common conditions	
Exacerbation of chronic bronchitis	Amoxicillin 500 mg po tds or doxycycline 200 mg on first day then 100 mg po daily (Doxycycline must not be used in pregnancy)
Community acquired pneumonia	Amoxycillin 500 mg po tds. Add clarithromycin 500 mg po BD if atypical organism suspected Doxycycline if penicillin allergy
Urinary tract infection	Trimethoprim 200 mg po BD. Nitrofurantoin 50 mg po QDS. If systemically unwell co-amoxiclav 375 mg po TDS
Cellulitis	Amoxycillin 500 mg po TDS plus flucloxacillin 500 mg po QDS, or clindamycin 450 mg po QDS (if penicillin allergy)
Suspected streptococcal tonsillitis	Phenoxymethyl penicillin 600 mg QDS

Minor Injury and Minor Illness at a Glance, First Edition. Edited by Francis Morris, Jim Wardrope, and Shammi Ramlakhan.

Plan

Advice

Patients want to know what is wrong with them. Often there is a clear diagnosis but in many cases there is significant doubt.

• *Clear diagnosis.* For example 'You have a broken leg'.

• *Probable diagnosis.* A specific diagnosis is likely but there is some room for doubt: 'You have tonsillitis. This is most likely due to a viral infection. Let us try simple treatments and it should get better in a few days, but if your symptoms get worse, or if you vomit, then come back or see GP.'

• *No diagnosis, diagnosis not time critical.* At times there is no clear diagnosis; for example, over 50% of patients admitted to hospital with abdominal pain will end up with a diagnosis of 'nonspecific abdominal pain'. In such cases, if you are discharging a patient, then say 'It is not clear what is causing your pain. There are no signs of a serious condition at present but things can change. If things get no better/worse or if new symptoms develop then come back or seek medical advice.'

• *No diagnosis, serious pathology needs ruled out.* There are some conditions, such as chest pain or sudden severe headache, where you have to go to some lengths to exclude a serious condition as any deterioration could be very sudden.

Medication

• *Over-the-counter drugs.* There is a large variety of drugs available without prescription. Paracetamol is a very effective analgesic and reduces fever quickly. Just because a drug is widely available does not mean it is less effective. If a drug is needed for a minor illness or injury, then over-the-counter drugs should be first-line management.

• *Prescription-only drugs.* The most common prescription-only drugs used in the treatment of minor illness and injury are antibiotics or second-line analgesics (Table 2.1). Specific guidance will be given in each of the sections of the book if drugs are indicated.

Physical treatments (exercise, physiotherapy, walking aids)

In musculo-skeletal problems and minor injuries, advice on physical treatment is vital. For example, in simple low mechanical back pain there is good evidence from controlled clinical trials that mobilisation and 'trying to keep going' result in a quicker recovery than rest. Joint function depends so much on the 'dynamic stabilisers' of good muscle tone and reflexes that periods of immobility can make a condition worse. The back muscles have to resist large forces due to the effects of the long lever (Figure 2.1).

Clearly, there are some conditions where immobilisation of a limb is required (e.g. significant fracture). If you advise a period of rest, then make arrangements for patient review.

Communications/advice (Figure 2.2)

• *Notes.* Good clinical notes are essential. Your assessment may be the first part of the patient's journey. Those who treat the patient need to know your findings, the results of tests and your initial diagnoses and treatment plans. If you have made good notes it is much easier to counter any complaint or litigation. Remember that clinical notes need to be signed, timed and dated each and every time that they are created and updated.

• *Communication with patient.* See 'Follow-up and safety net'. In some conditions it is essential to give written advice (e.g. if discharging a patient with a minor head injury).

• *Communication with carers.* Carers of young children, the elderly and those with learning disabilities need to be given the advice and instructions given to the patient.

• *Communication with other health professionals.* If you are referring a patient to another health professional then try to communicate your findings and the reason for referral. This may need a telephone call, a fax or a letter given to the patient (Figure 2.2).

• *Follow-up and safety net.* As a minimum, tell the patient to seek medical advice if their symptoms get worse or new symptoms develop. In certain conditions some symptoms are known as 'red flags', symptoms that indicate potentially serious pathology. Examples include the development of bladder or bowel symptoms in back pain (Figure 2.3).

⚑ Diagnoses not to be missed

Arriving at the correct diagnosis is the result of synthesis of information obtained from a good history, and examination and, where appropriate, investigations. The pitfalls in making a correct diagnosis and creating an appropriate management plan are:

• inadequate history
• inadequate history
• inadequate history
• ignoring abnormal vital signs (early-warning score)
• misuse/ poor interpretation of investigations
• closed thinking – too narrow differential diagnosis
• poor communication with patient
• no safety-net advice
• poor communication with other health professionals
• poor notes.

3 Wounds

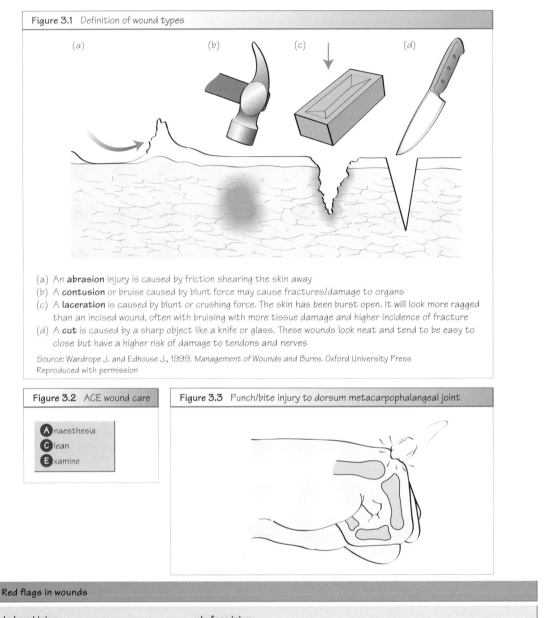

Figure 3.1 Definition of wound types

(a) An **abrasion** injury is caused by friction shearing the skin away
(b) A **contusion** or bruise caused by blunt force may cause fractures/damage to organs
(c) A **laceration** is caused by blunt or crushing force. The skin has been burst open. It will look more ragged than an incised wound, often with bruising with more tissue damage and higher incidence of fracture
(d) A **cut** is caused by a sharp object like a knife or glass. These wounds look neat and tend to be easy to close but have a higher risk of damage to tendons and nerves

Source: Wardrope J. and Edhouse J., 1999. Management of Wounds and Burns. Oxford University Press Reproduced with permission

Figure 3.2 ACE wound care

Anaesthesia
Clean
Examine

Figure 3.3 Punch/bite injury to dorsum metacarpophalangeal joint

Red flags in wounds

In hand injury
- Damage to tendon and nerve
- Fractures in crush injury
- Punch (human bite) injury to dorsum metacarpophalangeal joint
- High pressure injection injury

In face injury
- Cosmetic issues especially wounds of eyelids and vermillion border lip
- Damage to facial nerve and parotid duct

In wound infection
- Patients with systemic signs of infection (temperature, tachycardia, rigors)
- Patients with severe pain and signs of wound infections (necrotising fasciitis)
- Diabetic foot infections

Approach to the patient
History

• *Mechanism of injury* (Figure 3.1). *Glass and knife* wounds cut to the bone. *Crush injuries* cause more local tissue damage and fractures. *Penetrating injury* may harbour a foreign body, result in damage to deep structures. *Bites* carry infection risks. *Assaults/non-accidental* wounds have legal or safeguarding issues. *Self-inflicted* wounds also need a psychiatric assessment.

• *Time since injury.* Long delays to wound cleaning (more than 6h) means a higher risk of infection.

• *Past medical history.* Diabetes (neuropathy/infection), warfarin (bleeding), allergy, tetanus immunisation status.

Minor Injury and Minor Illness at a Glance, First Edition. Edited by Francis Morris, Jim Wardrope, and Shammi Ramlakhan.

Examination

Examine the *wound* – type (cut/laceration/abrasion/penetrating), site, size and depth; examine *structures deep to wound* – tendon and nerve function, vascular supply, bony injury and joint injury.

Investigations

X-ray for glass and possible bony injury, ultrasound for wood foreign body, bacteriology for infected wounds, and INR if the patient is taking warfarin and bleeding is a problem.

Documentation

A picture (or diagram) is worth many words. Note size/shape/surrounding features. Record distal sensation/nerve function/vascular status. Record past medical history/drugs/allergy.

Wound treatment

- *ACE wound care* (Figure 3.2):
  - **A**naesthesia may not be required for all wounds but greatly assists proper wound cleaning and examination.
  - **C**leaning is the most important part of wound care. Remove all dirt. Most contamination is easily removed using swabs, but scissors or a scrubbing brush may be required. The wound should be washed out with large volumes of fluid; a running tap is a good method.
  - **E**xamine the wound closely, especially incised wounds, to check for damage to deep structures and to check all dirt has been removed.
- *Wound closure.* Some wounds are best left open or referred to the emergency department for care:
  - wounds more that 6–12 h old – infection risk
  - bites – especially to the hand
  - infected wounds – do not try to close these.
  - heavily contaminated wounds
  - severe crush injury
  - evidence of damage to deeper structures.

  There are many ways to close wounds, each has its advantages and disadvantages:
  - *Sutures and staples* are good for control of bleeding, for gaping wounds and wounds across joints and hands.
  - *Glue* is effective for facial wounds (not eyelid or lips).
  - *Adhesive strips* are easy to apply, do not tear out and do not interfere with blood supply. Used for pretibial lacerations and small face wounds (not effective on bleeding wounds).
- *Tetanus immunisation.* Tetanus is a completely preventable disease that kills hundreds of thousands of people worldwide each year. The spores of tetanus are everywhere, but risks are greater in wounds contaminated by soil or manure, puncture wounds and deep wounds, especially if there is tissue damage. If a wound is judged to be at high risk of tetanus, then tetanus immunoglobin should be given and a tetanus toxoid booster if required.
- *Rabies.* Very rare in the UK, but think of this diagnosis if the bite occurred abroad. Refer all animal bites sustained abroad for assessment of rabies risk.
- *Antibiotics.* Antibiotics are not required for most wounds. The best way to reduce infection is 'ACE' wound care. Absolute indications would be evidence of a spreading infection, compound fractures and human bites. They might be required in some dog bites and some puncture wounds (e.g. feet).

Specific wounds

Hand wounds

The hand is a key sensory and motor organ (try wearing a bandage on your thumb for a day). Even minor wounds can cause significant disability. Take care in assessment. Ask the patient their occupation and hobbies and if they are right or left handed.
- Cuts caused by glass or knives often cause tendon or nerve injury.
- Crush injuries often cause fractures.
- Severe finger dislocations can cause lacerations.
- Beware the 'knuckle sandwich', a wound to the back or the hand over the metacarpal heads caused by punching a tooth, high infection risk and high risk of joint penetration (Figure 3.3).
- High-pressure injection injuries cause major tissue damage.

Facial wounds

Cosmetic implications should always be considered, but most can be managed by good wound care.
- Lip injury – cuts involving the vermillion border need careful closure. Ensure a laceration to a lip is not 'through and through' as this will need to be closed in layers.
- Deep wounds to the cheek can affect the parotid duct and/or one of the five branches of the facial nerve.
- Wounds that cross the margin of the eyelids need referral.
- X-rays of facial bones may be needed, especially in assault cases.

Pretibial lacerations

Rarely need suture. The shin has poor vascular supply, and even in the young these wounds have a tendency to ulcerate and may take months to heal. Adhesive strips, appropriate dressings and wool and crepe bandaging give the best results. If they are very deep or extensive, consider a plastic surgery opinion.

Bites

Extensive wound cleaning is the key to the prevention of infection. Wound should not be closed unless cosmetic appearance is a concern. Consider X-ray for tooth or fracture. Consider prophylactic antibiotic cover.

Needlestick

Wash the wound and ensure patient is immunised against tetanus and hepatitis B. If the 'source patient' is known and if they are high risk for HIV infection then refer urgently for consideration of HIV prophylaxis.

Wound infection

If localised signs of infection, then remove sutures, wash out and consider antibiotics. If there is more extensive erythema or lymphangitis, then remove sutures, wash out, antibiotics, review and follow up. If there is spreading infection or systemic symptoms (unwell, lymphangitis to axilla or groin, pyrexia, rigors), remove sutures, wash out, intravenous antibiotics and consider admission.

> ### ▶ Diagnoses not to be missed
>
> - *In diabetics*, always treat aggressively with good wound toilet and antibiotics. Refer all diabetic foot infections.
> - *Necrotising fasciitis* is characterised by excruciating pain. The local signs may be relatively innocuous in the early stages. Immediate referral for resuscitation and surgical treatment is required.

Box 4.1 Essential history

- On-set of symptoms
- Rate of progression
- Associated symptoms i.e. itchiness, discharge, pain
- Systemic upset – fever, rigors
- Immune status – diabetes, HIV, steroids
- Recent trauma/surgery
- Recent antibiotic therapy
- Foreign travel
- Animal exposure

Box 4.2 Examination

- Vital signs – temperature, blood pressure, pulse rate and blood sugar
- Anatomical site/distribution – with the site being marked to assess for spread of erythema
- Type of rash, e.g. raised, erythema, exudative, crusting, vesicular/bullous
- Skin colour
- Local lymphadenopathy
- Lymphangitis – erythema travelling up the lymphatic system
- Presence of gas under the tissues
- Evidence of precipitating breakdown of normal skin barriers, e.g. trauma or fungal infection

Figure 4.1 Cellulitis

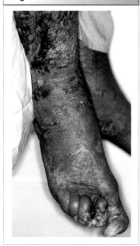

Figure 4.2 Erysipelas

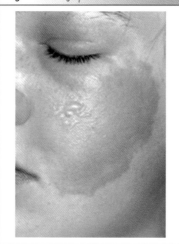

Figure 4.3 Impetigo

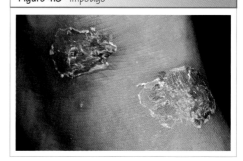

Figure 4.5 A boil

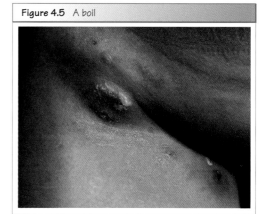

Figure 4.4 Folliculitis

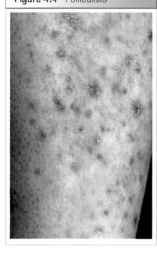

Figure 4.2: *Source*: Burns T, Breathnach S, Cox N & Griffiths C (2010) *Rook's Textbook of Dermatology*, 8th edn. Reproduced with permission of John Wiley & Sons Ltd.

All other photographs: *Source*: Buxton P & Morris-Jones R (2010) *ABC of Dermatology*, 5th edn. Reproduced with permission of John Wiley & Sons Ltd.

Figure 4.6 Formation of a cutaneous abscess and treatment

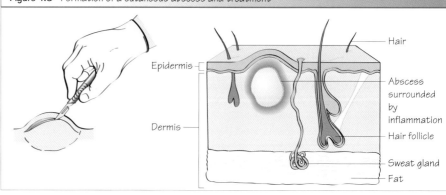

Hair
Epidermis
Abscess surrounded by inflammation
Dermis
Hair follicle
Sweat gland
Fat

Minor Injury and Minor Illness at a Glance, First Edition. Edited by Francis Morris, Jim Wardrope, and Shammi Ramlakhan.

Soft tissue infections can present in a number of different ways and in many different areas of the body. Most patients are systemically well; however, it is essential to recognise those patients that require parenteral therapy.

Approach to the patient

A careful history is essential. Essential history (see Box 4.1) and thorough examination (Box 4.2) are required to arrive at the correct diagnosis.

Cellulitis and erysipelas

Cellulitis (Figure 4.1) is the inflammation of dermal and subcutaneous connective tissue caused by bacteria. It may be acute, sub-acute or chronic. **Erysipelas** (Figure 4.2) is inflammation of the dermis and the upper subcutaneous tissues and is considered a form of cellulitis, rather than a discrete entity.

Bacteriological testing is only positive in a quarter of cases, but the most common causative organisms are groups A and G haemolytic streptococci and *Staphylococcus aureus*. Typically, the condition is characterized by redness of the skin accompanied by pain and swelling. It can affect any area of the skin, but most commonly affects the lower limbs. Erysipelas classically is an area raised above surrounding tissue and there is clear demarcation between affected and unaffected skin.

Features of severe cellulitis include rapid progression of swelling, blistering and systemic upset. The mainstays of treatment are antibiotics and elevation of the affected limb (if applicable). Penicillinase-resistant penicillins or cephalosporins are usually the most appropriate antibiotic.

Impetigo

Impetigo (see Chapter 44) is a highly contagious infection, usually of exposed areas of skin such as the face, by beta-haemolytic streptococci +/− *S. aureus* (Figure 4.3). It tends to have the classical appearance of yellow fluid-containing vesicles/pustules that rupture to form a golden/brown crusting. Oral antibiotics, such as flucloxacillin, are the treatment of choice.

Cutaneous abscess

An **abscess** is defined as a collection of pus in the dermis and deeper skin tissues. Skin is a very good barrier to bacterial invasion. Breaks in the skin due to abrasions, bites and eczema can give rise to infection that, through necrosis and liquefaction, can lead to abscess formation. This tends to be surrounded by erythematous tissue. The infective organisms are often skin flora.

The only definitive treatment for an abscess is incision and adequate and thorough drainage. Care must be made to break down all loculations within the cavity and the wound should be left open to promote continued drainage of any residual septic material. Packing the cavity prevents premature closure and allows appropriate healing by secondary intention. In the case of large lesions, general anaesthesia may be required in the interest of completed drainage and patient comfort. Provided incision and drainage are performed correctly, oral antibiotics are only indicated in the presence of significant surrounding erythema or systemic symptoms.

An abscess resulting from a hair follicle penetrating the dermis is called a pilonidal abscess. They most commonly occur in the natal cleft and most will require formal drainage and exploration.

Furuncle and carbuncle

Staphylococcal hair follicle infection is common (**folliculitis**, Figure 4.4) and is often found on the face, neck, axilla and thighs. A **furuncle** (also termed a boil; Figure 4.5) is a more extensive infection at the base of a hair follicle with a connected suprative collection in the subcutaneous tissues. The causative organism is usually *S. aureus*. A **carbuncle** occurs when several furuncles in the same site contribute to a coalescing inflammatory mass with multiple points of pus drainage. This more commonly occurs in diabetic patients and can often be found on the nape of the neck.

In the majority of furuncles, application of warm, moist heat to the area is all that is required. This promotes drainage, and thus healing. Larger furuncles and all carbuncles require formal incision and drainage.

Incision and drainage

A cutaneous abscess or large carbuncle requires incision and drainage (Figure 4.6).

In suitable cases, informed consent should be obtained and the procedure explained to the patient. Provide your patient with adequate analgesia before onset of the procedure.

The area should be cleansed, draped and sterility maintained and the anaesthetic should be administered in a field block, being cautious to avoid inoculation of the abscess itself; incise the abscess along the length of the fluctuant area and be careful to break down any loculations within the abscess so that all the pus is drained; then pack the abscess and apply a simple dressing.

Hidradenitis suprativa

This distressing condition manifests as recurrent abscess formation in areas of the body bearing high concentrations of apocrine sweat glands, such as the axilla, breast, thigh, groin and buttocks. Abscess formation, which is often multiple, may require surgical drainage to relieve symptoms, and can be complicated by sinus formation, granulomatous tissue and bacterial infection of the deep structures and surrounding dermis.

Animal and human bite wounds

Animal bite wounds carry a high risk of developing purulence or abscess (up to 58% and 20% respectively, depending on the animal). The causative organisms are often mixed and consist of animal/human oral and host skin flora.

Cat bites carry a higher risk of osteomyelitis, abscess formation and septic arthritis as they have pointed hollow teeth, whereas dog bites tend to cause a greater degree of crush injury.

Human bite wounds tend to be occlusive wounds (the teeth enclose an area of tissue) or involve the knuckles of an assailant.

All bite wounds should be irrigated copiously and explored for potential retention of tooth fragments and damage to (and inoculation of) deeper structures, such as synovium, joint capsules, nerves and tendons. Oral amoxicillin/clavulanate is an often and appropriate oral antibiotic. Other options include doxycycline, fluroquinolones, cephalosporins and the addition of metronidazole.

As with all wounds, a patient's tetanus status needs to be considered. Also, do not forget the potential for rabies in wounds sustained abroad.

5 Other soft tissue infections

Figure 5.1 Cold sore

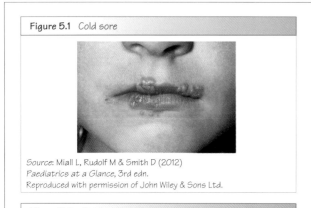

Source: Miall L, Rudolf M & Smith D (2012)
Paediatrics at a Glance, 3rd edn.
Reproduced with permission of John Wiley & Sons Ltd.

Figure 5.3 Common herpes zoster sites

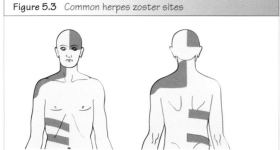
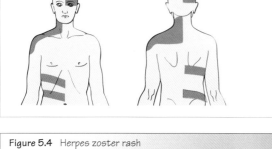
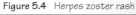

Figure 5.4 Herpes zoster rash

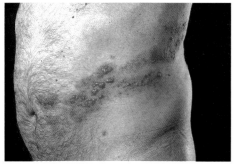

(a)
Source: Graham-Brown R & Burns T (2011)
Lecture Notes Dermatology, 10th edn.
Reproduced with permission of John Wiley & Sons Ltd.

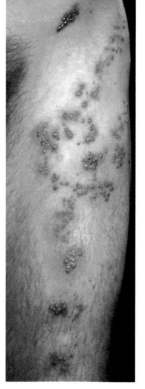

(b)
Source: Buxton P & Morris-Jones R (2010)
ABC of Dermatology, 5th edn.
Reproduced with permission of John Wiley & Sons Ltd.

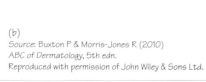

Figure 5.2 Chickenpox

Time in days		
	Macule	
2	Papule	
4	Fluid-filled vesicle	
6	Crusting	

Figure 5.5 Common scabies sites

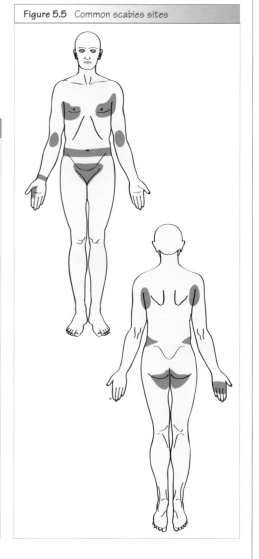

Viral soft tissue infection

Herpes simplex

Herpes simplex virus (HSV) is responsible for herpetic stomatitis and the recurrent form of the disease, herpes labialis (cold sore). These are primarily caused by HSV type-1; however, type-2 (genital herpes) can also give rise to these conditions. Primary infection is characterised by a preceding hyperaesthesia of the skin, followed by vesicle formation that progress onto painful ulceration. The virus then remains dormant, commonly in the trigeminal ganglia, and can be reactivated. This gives rise to the recurrent episodes most sufferer's experience.

Topical application of antiviral creams can limit the length of recurrence and reduce pain. There is no effective eradication therapy.

Varicella zoster

Varicella zoster virus (VZV) is responsible for the clinical manifestations known as **chickenpox** and **shingles** (herpes zoster). Chickenpox is the primary infection and tends to occur in childhood. It manifests as an initial pyrexial illness with myalgia and headache followed by macular to vesicular rash to the skin and mucosal surfaces. Spread is via direct contact or airborne spread. The individual remains highly contagious until all the vesicles have crusted over.

The illness is usually self-limiting and mild in childhood but can be extremely debilitating in adulthood. It is extremely rare to suffer a second bought of chickenpox. Treatment is generally supportive with antipyretics, such as paracetamol. The virus lays dormant in the dorsal root and cranial nerve ganglia and can present in later life as shingles.

Shingles is characterised by a preceding hyperaesthesia and pain in the dermatomal distribution of the dorsal nerve root involved. A rash similar in appearance to chickenpox then erupts in that dermatome. Shingles normally involves the trunk, is painful and develops over a number of days with crops of vescicles appearing and then crusting over. Ophthalmic zoster involves the forehead and eye and requires review by an ophthalmologist. Antiviral medication, such as acyclovir, can be used to reduce the duration of the illness and the risks of developing post-infective neuralgia.

Molluscum contagiosum

Molluscum contagiosum is a self-limiting viral skin infection. It is transmitted by direct skin-to-skin contact either by auto-inoculation or person-to-person contact and has an incubation period of 1–6 weeks. It is highly contagious and transmission is increased by wet skin.

Molluscum appears as umbilicated pearly or skin-coloured papules and can affect any part of the body. Mollusca usually last around 6 months and then undergo spontaneous regression but can last up to 2 years. Diagnosis is usually clinical and no treatment is required, although curette, cautery or cryosurgery can be used.

Fungal soft tissue infections

Tinea pedis is a fungal infection, more commonly known as athlete's foot, that occurs between the toes. It is itchy and can be persistent. The treatment is topical antifungal agents such as miconozole or clomitrazole. Breaks in the skin caused by athlete's foot can be the portal of entry for bacteria, giving rise to cellulitis as the usual protective barrier the skin provides is lost.

Candida albicans is a commensal of the mouth but can cause opportunistic infection of the skin. Predisposing factors include moist and opposing skin folds, immunosuppression (diabetes, etc.), obesity, poor hygiene and the use of broad-spectrum antibiotics.

The most common manifestation of *C. albicans* is genital thrush. This condition is a painful vulvovaginitis, characterised by white plaques and a white vaginal discharge. The condition can manifest orally, resulting in white plaque formation in the oral cavity, and can coexist with angular stomatitis.

Tinea capitis is a fungal infection of the scalp. It is caused by dermophyte invasion of the hair follicles. Features of the condition are areas of alopecia, which may be accompanied by erythema, pustule formation, scaling and itching. Peak incidence is amongst pre-adolescence, becoming rare after the age of 16. Males from African descent are most commonly affected. It is commonly **misdiagnosed as bacterial infection**. The treatment is oral griseofulvin (or similar antifungal agent) accompanied by selenium- or ketoconazole-based shampoo to prevent spread of the disease.

Insect bites

Insect bites can vary in their presentation depending on the causative organism. Lesions can vary from itchy wheals to large bullous lesions. They commonly present on the upper and lower limbs and the trunk. The cutaneous reaction, caused by inoculation or allergic reaction, is usually self-limiting. Common culprits include mosquitos, fleas, mites and ticks. Such bites may be the mode of transmission of significant diseases (malaria, Lyme disease and brucellosis). Insect bites can disrupt the skin's barrier to bacterial invasion, resulting in cellulitis around the area of the bite.

Infestations

Scabies is the term given to the skin eruptions (papules, vesicles, pustules and nodules) that arise from the burrows made by the mite *Sarcoptes scabiei*. These eruptions are extremely pruritc and arise as an immune response to the mite, its faeces and its eggs. It can be pandemic, and spread is via direct contact. Incubation is anywhere between 24h and 6 weeks. The areas most commonly affected are the hands/wrist, feet, ankles, genitalia, buttocks and abdomen. Diagnosis can be difficult, as finding a typical burrow can be obscured by scratching. Crusted scabies (Norwegian scabies) is a fulminant form of the condition found in immunocompromised and elderly patients.

Treatment of scabies is with the topical miticide permethrin and strict personal hygiene advice (not sharing towels, etc.).

> ### ▶ Diagnoses not to be missed
>
> #### Necrotising fasciitis
>
> Necrotising fasciitis is a rapidly progressing infection of the subcutaneous tissues spreading along the superficial fascial planes. Often arising from a trivial skin lesion, it may resemble cellulitis initially, but the pain is severe. Progression of infection is extremely rapid. Systemic toxicity with high temperatures and features of sepsis quickly follow. Most cases are polymicrobial; however, commonly isolated pathogens are *Streptococcus pyogenes* and *Staphylococcus aureus*.
>
> Necrotising fasciitis carries an extremely high mortality, and if suspected requires aggressive resuscitation, urgent and often multiple surgical debridements and broad-spectrum antibiotics initiated after discussion with a microbiologist.
>
> Fournier's gangrene is the eponymous name given to necrotising fasciitis of the perineum.

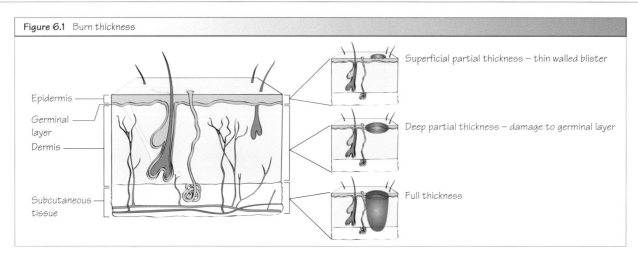

Figure 6.1 Burn thickness

Epidermis

Germinal layer

Dermis

Subcutaneous tissue

Superficial partial thickness – thin walled blister

Deep partial thickness – damage to germinal layer

Full thickness

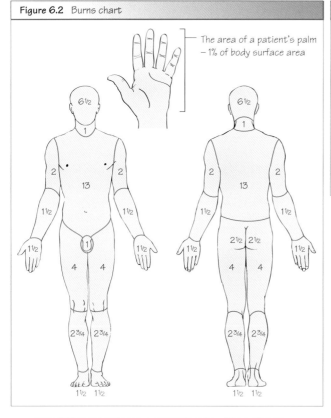

Figure 6.2 Burns chart

The area of a patient's palm – 1% of body surface area

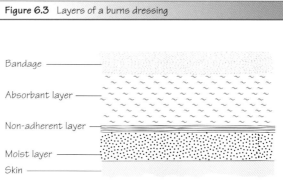

Figure 6.3 Layers of a burns dressing

Bandage

Absorbant layer

Non-adherent layer

Moist layer

Skin

Box 6.1 Indications for referral to burns specialist

- Superficial burns over more than 10% body surface area
- Age less than 5 years or more than 60 years
- Significant burns of the hand, face or perineum
- Full-thickness burns of the feet
- Circumferential burns
- Inhalational injury

Box 6.2 Signs of smoke inhalation

- Increased respiratory rate/dyspnoea
- Soot around nose and mouth
- Singeing of facial/nasal hair
- Soot in mouth
- Burns in and around mouth and nose

Red flags in burns

- Airway problems develop quickly after inhalation injury
- Think about carbon monoxide poisoning
- Large burns need referral
- Chemical burns often cause deep injury
- High voltage electrical burns cause deep tisue damage
- Think about non-accidental injury in vunerable groups

Minor Injury and Minor Illness at a Glance, First Edition. Edited by Francis Morris, Jim Wardrope, and Shammi Ramlakhan.

22 © 2014 John Wiley & Sons, Ltd. Published 2014 by John Wiley & Sons, Ltd. Companion Website: www.ataglanceseries.com/minorinjury

The key to correct burn management is to assess the depth of the injury and the percentage of the body surface area involved.

Burns are often described as superficial partial thickness, deep partial thickness or full thickness (Figure 6.1).

Approach to the patient

The history can give important clues. The depth of injury is proportional to the heat of the object/substance causing the burn and the contact time. Even relatively 'safe' heat sources such as domestic radiators can cause deep burns if there is a prolonged contact time. Some chemicals can cause very deep burns. Cement and hydrofluoric acid (used in industry for etching) cause major deep tissue destruction.

Conversely, most water scalds cause superficial injury, unless the contact time is prolonged; for example, where clothing is soaked with boiling water it takes time to remove the clothing and this can result in a deep burn.

Examination helps in grading the depth. With a superficial burn the blister is thin walled, the underlying skin is pink/red and sensation is intact (these are often very painful). A full-thickness burn is white leathery and often relatively pain free. A deep partial-thickness burn blisters; the skin is often a darker red but sensation is preserved. All three grades of burn can exist in one injury: sometimes the centre of the burn is full thickness, grading out to superficial at the periphery.

The area of the burn is best assessed using a burns chart (see Figure 6.2), but an approximation can be made; the area of the patient's hand is approximately 1% of their surface body area.

The part of the body involved is also important in the assessment. Burns of the hands, face, eyes and perineum may need special treatment.

Burns and scalds in children, the elderly and vulnerable adults may have been caused non-accidentally.

Assessment

Note the mechanism of burning. How hot was the source? Was contact time prolonged? Was there any exposure to fumes? Were there any other injuries? Note past medical history, drugs, tetanus immunisation status and allergy.

Assess the size and depth of the burn. If there has been exposure to smoke or flames, examine the mouth and nose for signs of burning/hair singeing or soot.

Treatment

Most small burns and scalds are suitable for outpatient treatment. The criteria for discussion with a burns specialist are listed in Box 6.1. First-aid treatment requires removal of the burning agent. This has usually been done before the patient attends, but in chemical burns it is safer to wash the area with large volumes of water. Cling film is an excellent temporary dressing and it also helps a great deal with pain relief.

Dealing with burn blisters

If the blisters are intact then they may be left (unless they are so thin walled that it is clear they will burst very soon). The blister reduces the incidence of infection and also helps pain relief.

Burns may be treated by exposure to the air or dressed. Most of the time a dressing is best; exceptions would be burns of the face and of the perineum.

The aim of a burns dressing is to provide a moist environment to help healing, with a dry adsorbent layer above this to soak up any exudate and then a layer to hold the dressing in place (see Figure 6.3). The dressing may be left in place for 5 days unless the bandages become soaked in exudate, when the outer layers should be replaced.

Most minor burns will heal in 5–10 days.

Ensure the patient is immunised against tetanus. Prophylactic antibiotics are *not* used.

Deep burns

The principles of management are the same, but it is best to discuss management and follow-up with a burns unit. Sometimes it can be hard to assess the depth of a burn on the initial attendance. Review in 3–5 days may make this judgement easier.

Burns in special areas

• *Hands.* Superficial scalds can be treated in a plastic bag. Deep burns should be referred early.
• *Face.* Check for signs of smoke inhalation. Check for corneal burns by instilling fluoroscein. Most superficial burns can be treated by exposure.
• *Perineum.* Difficult to dress and high infection risk. Refer.

Special types of burn

• *Chemical.* The commonest chemical burn is from cement (lime is a very strong alkali). These burns are often deep partial or full thickness). Brush off any powder and then wash with large amounts of water. Hydrofluoric acid causes penetrating burns. Use calcium gluconate gel and refer.
• *Electrical.* These are often deep burns. Small contact burns from domestic supply can be treated conservatively. High-voltage electricity travels up a limb through nerves, bone and muscle. The internal tissue damage can be greater than the skin burns. Always refer these burns.

> ### Diagnoses not to be missed
>
> #### Smoke inhalation and carbon monoxide poisoning
>
> Most deaths from house fires are caused by fumes. Hot gases can cause burns to the airway. If there are signs of smoke inhalation then the airway must be assessed and if necessary secured by endotracheal intubation. See Box 6.2 for the signs of smoke inhalation.
>
> In any patient exposed to a fire in a confined space, check the carbon monoxide level. Carbon monoxide binds to haemoglobin, reducing the oxygen-carrying capacity of the blood. Significant toxicity is unlikely with levels below 10% (unless there has been a significant time since burning and the patient has been treated with oxygen). Unconscious patients or those with neurological signs should be discussed with a hyperbaric oxygen centre.

7 Head injury and transient loss of consciousness

Figure 7.1 Glasgow coma scale

Eyes		Motor		Verbal	
Open spontaneously	4	Obeys verbal commands	6	Orientated in time/place/person	5
Open to voice	3	Localises to pain	5	Confused conversation	4
Open to pain	2	Flexion–withdrawal	4	Inappropriate sounds	3
No response	1	Flexion abnormal	3	Incomprehensible sounds	2
		Extension	2	No response	1
		No response	1		

Box 7.1 Indications for CT scan in patients with head injury

- Amnesia of > 30 min pre-injury
- History of loss of consciousness and age > 65 or dangerous mechanism of injury
- Reduced GCS
- New confusion
- Vomiting > 1 in an adult, > 3 times in a child
- Focal neurological signs
- Signs of basal skull fracture (panda eyes, bleeding from ears, CSF from nose, bruising over mastoid process)
- Taking warfarin/other anticoagulant

Box 7.2 Head injury discharge instructions

Should have responsible adult at home to observe. Return if:
- Persistent vomiting
- Worsening/severe headache
- Reduction in level of consciousness

Box 7.3 Indications for further invstigations

After a non-traumatic loss of consciousness refer the following for further assessment:
- An ECG abnormality
- Heart failure
- LOC on exertion
- Family history of sudden cardiac death in young
- An inherited cardiac condition
- > 65 years with no prodromal symptoms
- New breathlessness
- A heart murmur

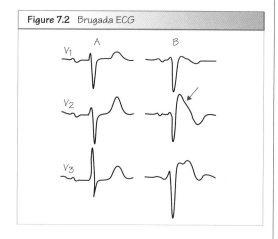

Figure 7.2 Brugada ECG

Minor Injury and Minor Illness at a Glance, First Edition. Edited by Francis Morris, Jim Wardrope, and Shammi Ramlakhan.

Head injury

Over 1 million patients with a head injury attend emergency departments every year. The great majority of these injuries do not result in serious complications. However, intracranial bleeding can have catastrophic consequences and so these patients need careful assessment.

Approach to the patient

History

• *Details of incident.* Certain mechanisms of injury, such as falls from a height or down stairs, road traffic accidents and assaults, increase the likelihood of serious problems. Some types of direct blow (object falling from a height onto head, hammer/golf club blows) increase the incidence of skull fracture. If there is no definite mechanism of injury, has there been a collapse that led to the injury? Has there been a loss of consciousness (LOC)? If so, for how long? Was there a period of loss of memory before or after the incident? Were alcohol or drugs consumed?

• *Past history.* Does the patient take warfarin or other anticoagulant? Are they alcohol dependent? Do they have other medical problems? Is there a history of pre-existing confusion that may lead to difficulty in assessing the level of consciousness?

• *Social history.* Do they have someone at home who can observe them if they are discharged?

Examination

Consider if the patient has any signs of a neck injury or if the mechanism of injury requires immobilisation of the neck.

There are four components to the examination of an uncomplicated minor head injury:

• *Level of consciousness.* Assess the Glasgow coma score (GCS) (Figure 7.1). Any reduction in the GCS is highly significant. Is the person orientated in time, place and person?

• *Vital signs.* Check pulse and blood pressure.

• *Examine the head.* Note any bruising, swelling, lacerations. In assault cases it is especially important to make detailed notes of wounds. Large scalp wounds, especially to the back of the head, can be missed; make sure you examine the whole of the scalp. Check nose and ears for bleeding or leaking of cerebrospinal fluid (CSF). See the chapter on facial injury/nose injury/mouth injury for examination of these areas.

• *Mini-neurological examination.* Where the patient is fully alert and with no worrying mechanism of injury then a brief neurological examination (5 × 5 × 5) should be carried out:

  ◦ *5 eye exams* – check papillary reactions, visual acuity and eye movements for diplopia and nystagmus.

  ◦ *5 face exams* – check facial movements and sensation, check ears for hearing/bleeding, check the tympanic membranes; *mouth* – look for injury and check tongue and palate movements. (See Chapter 8.)

  ◦ *5 limb exams* – check power (pronator drift), sensation, coordination (finger nose) and gait (heel to toe+normal gait – see Chapter 8), and reflexes.

Investigation

Most minor head injuries will need no investigation. The indications for computed tomography (CT) scan are shown in Box 7.1.

If suspicion of any neck injury, X-rays or CT may be required. If suspicion of bony injury to face or jaw, X-rays may be needed.

Management

• *Scalp lacerations.* These injuries can bleed profusely. Apply direct pressure and most bleeding will stop. Use lignocaine with adrenaline. If bleeding is profuse, get help. Use large mattress sutures through all layers of the wound.

• *Indications for observation.* Continued confusion or reduced GCS (with normal CT scan), continued vomiting or other neurological signs. Skull vault or base fracture with no complications.

• *Indications for neurosurgical advice.*
  ◦ Abnormal CT scan
  ◦ GCS deteriorating
  ◦ GCS <8.

• *Discharge instructions.* See Box 7.2.

• *Home with written and verbal advice.* A judgement has to be made if there is no adult who can observe the patient at home.

Transient loss of consciousness (no trauma)

Transient LOC with no history of head injury is a very common symptom. By far the commonest cause is a simple faint (vaso-vagal). This is usually a reaction to a painful or frightening situation where the heart rate is slowed, blood pressure drops, the patient is pale, clammy, feels sick and dizzy and then has a transient LOC. The other common problem is postural hypotension, especially in the elderly. However, there are some serious and potentially life-threatening problems that present in this way.

• *History.* Try to identify a trigger for a vaso-vagal. Was there a prodrome or was there no warning? Were there other symptoms, such as headache/chest pain or shortness of breath? Was it related to a sudden change in posture or prolonged standing? Was it related to exercise? Was there tongue biting or incontinence? Is there a previous history? Any family history? Was there any unilateral weakness? Is the patient taking any medications?

• *Exam.* Perform a general exam. Check vital signs, including lying and standing blood pressure. Specifically check for heart murmurs and neurological signs.

• *Investigation.* Perform an electrocardiogram (looking for conduction defects, bradycardias, tachycardia, signs of long/short QT, Brugada syndrome (Figure 7.2). Check blood sugar.

• *Management.* If typical vaso-vagal then reassure. Box 7.3 lists those that need further investigation.

► **Diagnoses not to be missed**

Cardiac syncope – aortic stenosis, complete heart block and arrthymias are all increasingly common with advancing age.

Therefore, in the middle-aged and elderly take a full history, e.g. ischaemic heart disease, exertional syncope, examine for murmurs (aortic stenosis) and carefully scrutinise the electrocardiogram.

Cardiac syncope in young person (exertional, family history, Brugada).

---

8 Neurological problems

Figure 8.2 Time is brain. FAST test: **Face** movements, **Arm** movements, **Speech**, **Time** is brain

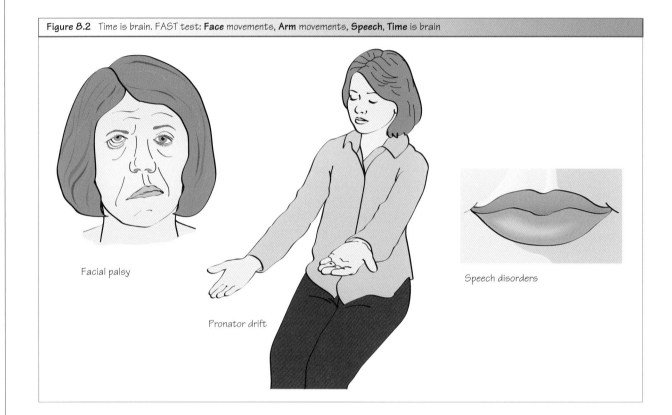

Facial palsy

Pronator drift

Speech disorders

Table 8.1 Common mononeuropathies

Symptom	Nerve	Common causes (less common)
Facial palsy	Facial nerve	Bell's palsy (Ramsay Hunt, stroke)
Wrist drop	Radial nerve	Saturday night palsy, trauma
Carpal tunnel syndrome	Median	Compression, trauma, pregnancy
Ulnar nerve palsy	Ulnar	Compression/trauma at elbow, compression at wrist (cycling)
Meralgia paraesthetica	Lateral cutaneous nerve thigh	Compression, obesity
Foot drop	Common peroneal	Compression, trauma, direct blow

Minor Injury and Minor Illness at a Glance, First Edition. Edited by Francis Morris, Jim Wardrope, and Shammi Ramlakhan.

Focal neurological deficit

- *History.* A good history is essential. The onset of symptoms is especially important. Are there other neurological symptoms, such as headache, nausea, vomiting, vertigo? Is there any preceding trauma? Systemic symptoms such as fever, vomiting, neck pain and photophobia are 'red flags'. Note the past medical history, especially of neurological problems, cancer, vascular problems. Check drug history, especially if taking anticoagulants.
- *Examination.* Carry out the FAST test, AMT and a $\times 5 \times 5 \times 5 \times 5$ brief neurological examination (Figure 8.1).

Time is brain

The advent of thrombolysis for thrombotic stroke means that any new focal neurological deficit needs very prompt assessment. Patients who are FAST-test positive (Figure 8.2) should be referred immediately for a computed tomography (CT) scan. **Always check the blood glucose**. Exceptions would be patients with a clear diagnosis of Bell's palsy or lesions due to peripheral nerve damage/compression/neuropathy (see later).

Acute confusion

The differential diagnosis is wide, but main causes are systemic upset (infection, hypoxia, hypoglycaemia, low blood pressure), intracranial problems (trauma/vascular/infection/tumour), drug/toxin related (alcohol, misuse of drugs, withdrawal), psychiatric causes.

- *History.* A good history is essential, but the patient may not be able to give a clear account, so seek details from family/friends/carers. Was the onset sudden or gradual? Any symptoms of infection, such as fever, local symptoms of infection headache, drug use or previous history?
- *Examination.* Always check vital signs. Does the patient look ill? Is there a rash? Any signs of local infection in the chest? Is the patient orientated in time, place and person (normal in most psychiatric causes)? Are there any neurological signs?
- *Investigation.* Always check the blood glucose, and it is prudent to strip test the urine. Otherwise the investigation will depend on the suspected causes.
- *Management.* This will depend upon the cause. **Do not assume confusion to be due to the effects of alcohol or drugs until other causes have been excluded**.

Fits

These are at times frightening events both for the patient and those caring for them. The vast majority of fits stop on their own, and the priority is to ensure safety and to prevent aspiration.

Manage patients on their side during a seizure and do not force anything into their mouth. It is normal for the patient to be confused for up to 30 min following a seizure.

Fit in a patient known to suffer from epilepsy

Injuries such as head lacerations and shoulder injuries may need hospital assessment, as will patients with prolonged or multiple seizures.

First fit

If the patient is not known have fits then they need a full assessment, including history, examination, vital signs and glucose measurement. They may need a CT scan. If they have made a complete recovery and there are no features to suggest the fits are secondary to a serious condition they will need assessment in a first-fit clinic. They should not drive until that assessment has been made.

Neuropathy
Bell's palsy

The onset is usually sudden and the patient notices asymmetry when they smile or try to close their eyes. They might drool from the corner of the mouth and notice loss of taste. It is caused by pressure on the facial nerve, probably due to viral infection, and is a lower motor neurone palsy. It is common in young adults.

The muscles controlling the whole of one side of the face are weak. This includes the forehead, which does not wrinkle when the patient frowns (in upper motor neurone problems such as stroke the forehead still moves).

A typical case of Bell's palsy is treated with corticosteroid and follow-up arranged. Most cases recover.

Radial nerve palsy

A common history is that the patient wakes up having been drinking heavily the previous night and slept very soundly with the arm in an awkward position; hence the name 'Saturday night palsy'. The patient cannot extend the fingers and wrist. There are a number of other causes of radial nerve palsy, so patient should be given a splint for the wrist and follow-up arranged.

Common peroneal nerve palsy

Compression of this nerve over the fibular head gives rise to acute foot drop. It needs to be differentiated from foot drop associated with back pain (radiculopathy); splintage and follow-up is required.

Meralgia paraesthetica

Compression of the lateral cutaneous nerve of the thigh gives rise to an area of well-localised numbness to anterolateral aspect of the upper thigh. This is a benign and frequently self-limiting condition.

▶ Diagnoses not to be missed

Guillain–Barré is an acute neuropathy associated with progressive limb weakness that reaches its worst within 4 weeks. The weakness is both proximal and distal with loss of reflexes and associated with sensory symptoms but few signs. Immediate referral to a neurologist is required.

Table 9.1 Important causes of primary and secondary headache

Primary	Secondary
Tension-type headache	Subarachnoid haemorrhage
Migraine (with or without aura)	Temporal arteritis
Cluster headache	Benign or malignant space occupying lesion
	Stroke (ischaemic or haemorrhagic)
	Meningitis
	Acute glaucoma
	Medication overuse
	Herpes zoster

Table 9.2 Red flag symptoms; SIGN guidelines 2008

- New onset or change in headache and age >50 years
- Sudden onset or thunderclap headache
- New focal neurological symptoms
- Change in cognition or personality
- Impaired consciousness
- Abnormal neurological examination
- Change in usual frequency and character of headache
- Headache affected by change in posture
- Headache affected by physical exertion, valsalva or cough
- Jaw claudication or visual disturbance in a patient age >50 years
- Neck stiffness
- Fever
- New-onset headache in a patient with a known history of cancer
- New-onset headache in a patient known to have HIV infection

Table 9.3

Was it of sudden or gradual onset?
Was it unilateral or bilateral?
What was the nature of the pain? e.g. tight, pressing or throbbing?
What was the severity?
How did if affect their usual daily activity?
Where there any associated symptoms?

Figure 9.1 CT of a patient with extensive SAH

This non-contrast CT scan of the brain shows extensive (bright white) subarachnoid blood. There is an associated hydrocephalus, as demonstrated by enlargement of the ventricular system

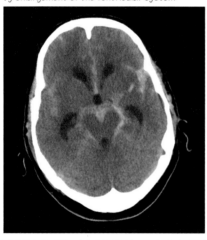

Figure 9.2 Contrast catheter angiogram

This angiogram demonstrates a large aneurysm of the anterior communicating artery

Headache accounts for 4% of primary care consultations. Migraine sufferers lose an average of two to three working days per year.

Approach to the patient

Broadly, headache can be divided into primary or secondary headache (Table 9.1). Recognise the 'red flag' symptoms that point towards a secondary cause for the headache and warrant further investigation. (Table 9.2).

Often a clear diagnosis can be made by taking an accurate history of the timing and duration of the symptoms, along with any associated or aggravating factors. When taking a history from a patient with headache, the questions in Table 9.3 will help point towards a diagnosis.

Minor Injury and Minor Illness at a Glance, First Edition. Edited by Francis Morris, Jim Wardrope, and Shammi Ramlakhan.

Take into account the age of the patient, as most of the secondary causes of headache are more common in the over-50 age group.

If the patient has recurrent symptoms, then a symptom diary may aid the diagnosis. It should include details of time and frequency, potential triggers, associated symptoms and, in women of childbearing age, relationship to menstruation.

A thorough neurological examination and blood pressure check is essential. Again, any abnormality would make a secondary cause for the headache more likely.

Common primary headaches
Tension-type headache
Tension-type headache is often described as a pressure or tight band-like headache. It is often bilateral and of gradual onset. It is usually mild to moderate in severity, with little effect on daily activity.

There is also a lack of the symptoms associated with migraine or cluster headache.

The treatment is with simple analgesia such as paracetamol or nonsteroidal anti-inflammatory drugs (NSAIDs).

Migraine
Migraine can be either unilateral or bilateral, is often described as a pulsating or throbbing headache and can last up to 72h. It is usually moderate to severe in severity and the patient will usually want to rest quietly when the headache is present. Nausea and vomiting can be associated symptoms, as can sensitivity to light and noise.

Some patients suffer migraine with aura. The patient may describe visual symptoms, such as flickering lights, or sensory symptoms such as pins and needles or numbness.

All of these symptoms should be fully reversible and typically last up to 1h. Occasionally, patients may suffer the aura without headache.

Further investigation should be considered if the aura is atypical (e.g. diplopia, motor weakness or reduced consciousness).

The treatment of an acute attack is with paracetamol, high-dose aspirin, NSAIDs and tryptans. Patients who are vomiting may require antiemetics and intravenous analgesia.

Cluster headache
Cluster Headache is a severe, unilateral headache often localised around the eye. It is associated with redness of the eye, watering of the eye and nasal congestion. There may also be some evidence of constriction of the pupil or sweating of the forehead. These symptoms are present on the same side as the headache. The symptoms last up to 4h and a good diagnostic test and the effective treatment is the administration of 100% oxygen.

Verapamil can be used as prophylaxis of cluster headache.

In general, it is important to remember that opiates should be avoided in the treatment of primary headache. Another point to consider is that overuse of analgesia may, in itself, cause a headache and should be considered in any patient presenting with chronic headache.

Secondary headache
Subarachnoid haemorrhage
Consider subarachnoid haemorrhage (SAH) in patients presenting with a sudden and severe headache. It is an important diagnosis not to be missed as a second bleed from an underlying cerebral aneurysm may be catastrophic. Typically, the headache reaches its maximum severity in seconds to minutes, is usually occipital and associated with nausea or vomiting and neck stiffness. These signs may be absent in up to 50% of patients with SAH.

An abnormal neurological examination will make the diagnosis of SAH more likely.

A computed tomography (CT) scan should be performed in the first instance and is most sensitive in the first 12h. The sensitivity declines rapidly with time. With CT scan alone around 6% of SAH will be missed (increasing further over time) (Figure 9.1). Therefore, a lumbar puncture should be performed in patients where SAH is suspected and the CT is normal.

Evidence of subarachnoid blood should prompt referral to the neurosurgical team for further management and investigation of an underlying vascular abnormality.

Temporal arteritis
Consider temporal arteritis or giant cell arteritis in patients over the age of 50, presenting with a throbbing unilateral or bilateral headache with scalp tenderness. There may be constitutional symptoms such as malaise, loss of appetite and weight loss. Other associated symptoms include jaw claudication, muscles pain and stiffness.

It can lead to sudden blindness caused by occlusion of the ophthalmic artery. The risks of myocardial infarction and stroke are also increased.

A raised erythrocyte sedimentation rate and C-reactive protein are typical and the diagnosis is made by histological examination of a temporal artery biopsy. The treatment is with high-dose corticosteroids and low-dose aspirin.

Infections
Sinusitis causes a frontal headache and facial pain, often described as a pressure or fullness. Sinusitis is often due to a viral infection, but may also be allergic or autoimmune in origin. It may be associated with an upper respiratory tract infection or a purulent nasal discharge. Typically the pain is worse on bending down. There may be some tenderness over the frontal and maxillary sinuses. First-line treatment is with steam inhalation, analgesia and decongestants. Antibiotics may be warranted if symptoms are severe or fail to settle in 7–10 days.

Frequently, mild constitutional headaches are associated with viral illnesses and upper respiratory tract infection. It is important not to miss bacterial meningitis, and this should be considered in anyone who presents with severe headache, fever and signs of meningism, such as photophobia and neck stiffness. Patients suspected to have bacterial meningitis should be assessed and treated promptly with intravenous antibiotics. The treatment of bacterial meningitis is beyond the scope of this chapter. Further information can be found at www.meningitis .org and your local hospital should have an appropriate antibiotic protocol.

Brain tumour
Consider a brain tumour in patients who present with headache and other signs of raised intracranial pressure, such as nausea, vomiting and altered consciousness. Approximately 50% of patients with a brain tumour report headache as the primary symptom. The headache is often worse in the morning and when bending down or straining. The diagnosis is made by imaging the brain with CT or magnetic resonance imaging and specialist referral.

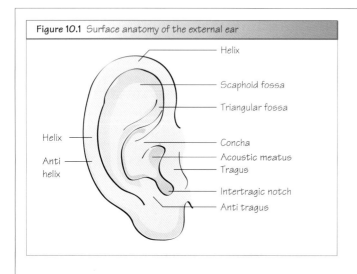

Figure 10.1 Surface anatomy of the external ear

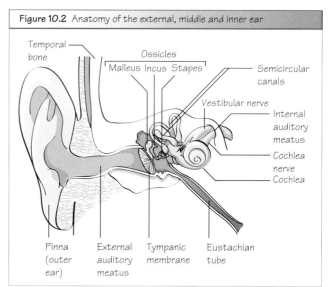

Figure 10.2 Anatomy of the external, middle and inner ear

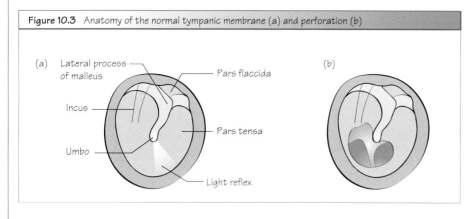

Figure 10.3 Anatomy of the normal tympanic membrane (a) and perforation (b)

Minor Injury and Minor Illness at a Glance, First Edition. Edited by Francis Morris, Jim Wardrope, and Shammi Ramlakhan.

30 © 2014 John Wiley & Sons, Ltd. Published 2014 by John Wiley & Sons, Ltd. Companion Website: www.ataglanceseries.com/minorinjury

Approach to the patient

The five cardinal symptoms to elicit when consulting a patient with potential ear problems are pain (otalgia), discharge, deafness/change of hearing, tinnitus and dizziness/vertigo.

Ear examination requires an otoscope with adequate positioning to the side of the patient. Start by inspecting the external ear (Figure 10.1), as well as the face, mouth, throat and neck. Next, palpate the pinna, especially the tragus, and mastoid and look for lymph nodes. Using the otoscope, inspect the external auditory canal and tympanic membrane (Figure 10.2). Hearing can be informally assessed by whispering or rubbing fingers together for each ear in turn. Formal tuning fork tests, Weber's and Rinne's tests, can also be performed (see Chapter 11).

Ear wax (cerumen impaction)

Cerumen glands provide a protective lipid layer. Impaction occurs though poor aural hygiene, and compounded through the use of cotton buds or water in the external auditory canal.

Symptoms are progressive hearing loss, acutely worsened if the wax has swollen due to water and a feeling of fullness to the ear. Pain is only present if cerumen is touching the tympanic membrane.

Treatment involves 2 weeks of olive oil applied topically to allow softening or the use of proprietary anti-wax eardrops and when required appropriate referral for ear syringing and repeat auroscopy and follow-up.

Otitis externa

Also known as *tropical ear* or *swimmer's ear*, this is an inflammatory infective condition affecting the external auditory canal. It results from bacteria, most commonly *Pseudomonas aeruginosa*, *Staphylococcus* and Gram-negative organisms, penetrating the protective lipid layer secreted by cerumen glands damaging the underlying squamous epithelial cells lining the external auditory canal. Otitis externa is common, affecting 1 in 10 people at some point during their lifetime.

Symptoms are pain with or without ear discharge and a painful fullness sensation to the ear itself. This is accentuated by jaw movement or traction on the ear pinna or by pressing on the tragus. The external auditory canal appears oedematous and erythematous with discharge evident.

Treatment is with topical combined antibiotics and steroids (e.g. Gentisone HC), and it is important to ensure that the tympanic membrane is intact before using these. Severe infection requires referral to ear, nose and throat (ENT) for irrigation and suction and antibiotic wick placement.

Otitis media

This is inflammation of the middle ear thought to be related to transient dysfunction of the Eustachian tube resulting in bacterial infection. *Haemophilus influenzae*, *Streptococcus pneumoniae* and *Moraxella catarrhalis* are the most common organisms.

Symptoms are typically acute onset otalgia with hearing disturbance.

Auroscopy shows bulging of the tympanic membrane with erythema.

Treatment with analgesia may be all that is required, as 80% improve spontaneously and only those persisting beyond 48 h require antibiotics.

Tympanic membrane perforation

This results in conductive hearing loss and may be caused by infection, trauma or iatrogeny (e.g. ear irrigation for cerumen removal) (Figure 10.3).

The presence of otalgia indicates a concurrent disease process.

The tympanic membrane will heal spontaneously even after multiple perforations; however, the presence of a perforation often allows infection to occur should water enter the external auditory canal.

Treatment involves avoiding water exposure to the affected ear. If concurrent infection is present, ototoxic topically applied ear drops should be *avoided*.

General practitioner/ENT follow-up should be arranged.

Foreign body

Foreign bodies in the ear canal are common and include toys, insects and most commonly cotton buds.

Some foreign bodies may be removed with irrigation, though others require crocodile forceps, or suction catheter.

Thorough examination is required post-removal to exclude residual or further foreign body and pre-existing iatrogenic injury.

If the foreign body is lying adjacent to the tympanic membrane or indeed has caused perforation or complete visualisation is not possible then removal should not be attempted and such patients should be referred to ENT.

Likewise, uncooperative patients, often children, should also be referred to ENT to avoid iatrogenic complications.

Patients may also present with foreign bodies to the ear lobe, such as a retained earring butterfly clip. These may require a local anaesthetic nerve block to achieve adequate analgesia for removal.

Acute hearing loss

Acute unilateral hearing loss is uncommon. The four main pathophysiological causes are viral-induced sensorineural hearing loss, immune-mediated sensorineural hearing loss, cochlea vascular compromise and intra-cochlea membrane rupture.

Patients therefore require a thorough ENT examination, a complete neurological examination especially focusing on the cranial nerves and cerebellar examination, as well as Rinne and Weber tests as outlined in Chapter 11.

Once wax is excluded, referral to ENT is required.

Wounds/lacerations to the ear

The external ear comprises an avascular cartilaginous skeleton covered by skin rich in blood supply, provided by the superficial temporal artery and posterior auricular artery.

Superficial skin lacerations may be closed with 5/0 or 6/0 non-absorbable sutures, taking care not to place the suture through the underlying cartilage. A pressure dressing around the head is helpful in preventing auricular haematoma formation. Sutures should be removed after 5 days with a wound check after 24 h to ensure the absence of auricular haematoma. Prophylactic antibiotics are advised.

Complex, contaminated wounds that involve the cartilage, partial amputation or those associated with auricular haematomas require referral.

▶ Diagnoses not to be missed

Acute mastoiditis

This is infection of the mastoid bone of the skull which presents with headache, pain, fever, systemic upset and erythema over the mastoid area. It is usually caused by an extension of acute otitis media.

Cholesteatoma

This is a tumour caused by growth of trapped squamous epithelium within the middle ear invading surrounding bone with compression and damage to adjacent structures. It presents with painless otorrhoea and progressive hearing loss and examination demonstrates tympanic membrane perforation with mucopurulent discharge and granulation tissue in the external auditory canal that persists despite antibiotics.

11 Dizziness and vertigo

Table 11.1 Peripheral and central vertigo

	Peripheral vertigo	Central vertigo
Onset	Sudden	Usually gradual
Systemic upset (e.g. nausea and vomiting)	Severe	Minimal
Nystagmus	Combined horizontal and rotary with inhibition by fixation on an object. Resolves within 48 h with fatigability on repeated testing. Unidirectional on movement	Purely vertical, horizontal or rotary, not inhibited by fixation on an object. Persisting beyond 48 h with no fatigue. Direction may change with gaze direction
Balance	Mild to moderate imbalance	Severe imbalance
Auditory symptoms (e.g. hearing loss, tinnitus)	Common	Rare
Effect of head position	Worsened by position	Persistent across all positions

Many patients complain of 'dizziness' which affects around 5% of the adult population per year. It is important to try to reach an accurate diagnosis as it is often a poorly understood area.

Dizziness is a lay term that patients use indiscriminately to describe a multitude of symptoms. It can be divided into vertiginous and non-vertiginous pathologies, as dizziness in itself is not a diagnosis.

The definition of vertigo is an illusion of movement, spinning, oscillating, and so on of either the patient or their environment due to pathology of the vestibular system or the cerebral processing of its information. This is in contrast to non-vertiginous presentations such as presyncope (a sensation of imminent faint or loss of conscious), light headedness (e.g. when standing up due to postural hypertension) and disequilibrium (altered gait/balance without head symptoms present).

True vertigo must be differentiated into central or peripheral origin (Table 11.1), as this dictates subsequent management.

Central vertigo is due to pathology of the central nervous system, most commonly caused by a stroke, multiple sclerosis, infection, trauma and acoustic neuroma, and such patients will invariably need radiological imaging.

Peripheral vertigo, meanwhile, is caused by pathology within the inner ear or vestibular system, with the most common causes being benign paroxysmal positional vertigo, Ménière's disease, labyrinthitis, visual vertigo and vestibular neuronitis.

Minor Injury and Minor Illness at a Glance, First Edition. Edited by Francis Morris, Jim Wardrope, and Shammi Ramlakhan.

Approach to the patient

A thorough history covering the points in Box 11.1 is essential.

A full systemic examination is required, with particular reference to the cardiovascular system (vascular disease/atrial fibrillation), the neurological examination (cranial nerve palsy, abnormal cerebellar signs, abnormal gait, limb weakness/hemiparesis) and the ear examination (tympanic membrane perforation, hearing loss, and Rinne and Weber tests).

Laboratory investigations aid little in the diagnosis of vertigo, which is a clinical diagnosis. For central vertigo, radiological imaging by computed tomography (CT) or magnetic resonance imaging (MRI) is essential.

Vestibular neuronitis

This is the commonest cause of a first episode of sustained vertigo. As it is not clearly inflammatory it is often referred to as a vestibular neuropathy. It is of unknown aetiology, most commonly occurring in middle-aged adults. Patients complain of a spontaneous sudden onset of severe vertigo with marked nausea and vomiting which persists for longer than 24 h.

Physical examination reveals a unidirectional spontaneous horizontal nystagmus which may be positional, with the fast phase towards the healthy ear. It may be terminated by visual fixation.

The Romberg test is positive, with the patient falling towards the pathological side.

Ear examination and the Rinne and Weber tests are normal, which distinguishes this from labyrinthitis.

The head impulse test, which tests for normal ocular fixation during rapid passive head rotation, is also abnormal.

Anti-emetics and vestibular suppressants are the mainstays of treatment, with patients requiring admission for severe symptoms. Recognised vestibular suppressants include low-dose benzodiazepines.

Antihistamines, such as cyclizine and cinnarizine, which have antimuscarinic and anti-emetic properties, are also ideal. Prochlorperazine is also particularly useful; however, medication should be limited to short-term use, with patients encouraged to mobilise as soon as possible.

Labyrinthitis

Labyrinthitis, compared with vestibular neuronitis, often presents with hearing loss and tinnitus. It is a viral-induced inflammation of the inner ear often following an upper respiratory tract infection. Other causes are bacterial infection, head injury, drugs or autoimmune.

Recovery typically takes up to 6 weeks, with some residual symptoms lasting much longer if permanent damage has occurred. Treatment again involves vestibular suppressants, and there is growing evidence that selective serotonin reuptake inhibitors may be more successful, as well as early antivirals and steroids.

Bacterial labyrinthitis requires antibiotics and referral to ear, nose and throat. Patients with chronic symptoms require vestibular rehabilitation.

Ménière's disease

This is idiopathic but is believed to be caused by an excess of endolymphatic fluid. Classical Ménière's is considered to have four classical symptoms: aural fullness or pressure in one or both ears; unilateral or bilateral tinnitus; fluctuating, progressive, unilateral or bilateral hearing loss typically in the lower frequencies; peripheral vertigo symptoms.

The Rinne test will be normal and the Weber test will be abnormal localising to the normal unaffected ear.

Management includes dietary modification, in particular tobacco, alcohol and caffeine avoidance and low salt intake.

Antihistamines and other anti-emetics are also used, as well as betahistine, which is the only drug to prevent symptoms by causing vasodilatation of the inner ear.

Benign paroxysmal positional vertigo

This is very common, due to the dislodgement of calcium crystals in the inner ear. It causes peripheral vertigo symptoms typically lasting only seconds to minutes and can only be induced by a change in head position. The diagnosis is clinical and can be confirmed by performing the Dix–Hallpike test and treated with the Epley manoeuvre.

Migraine

Central or peripheral vertigo features occur in up to 25% of patients suffering from acute migrainous vertigo. It is typified by migrainous-type headaches often with marked nausea and vomiting. Patients often prefer a darkened room owing to photophobia. There is also often a strong family history of migraine.

Vestibular schwannoma

Vestibular schwannoma, often termed acoustic neuroma, is a benign intracranial tumour of the myelin-forming cells of the vestibulocochlear nerve. Incidents peak in the fifth and sixth decades of life.

Early signs and symptoms are ipsilateral sensorineural hearing loss/deafness which is progressive, with 80% of patients also complaining of tinnitus. Vertiginous symptoms are rare because of chronic central compensation.

 Diagnoses not to be missed

Cerebellar stroke/transient ischaemic attack

Isolated vertigo is unlikely to be the result of cerebral vascular disease unless it is associated with other neurological brain stem symptoms or signs (e.g. ataxia, dysarthria, diplopia, headache).

It typically affects older patients with hypertension, diabetes, ischaemic heart disease, hypercholesterolaemia and previous stroke or transient ischaemic attack.

Onset of symptoms is sudden and confirmation of the diagnosis is made on CT or MRI.

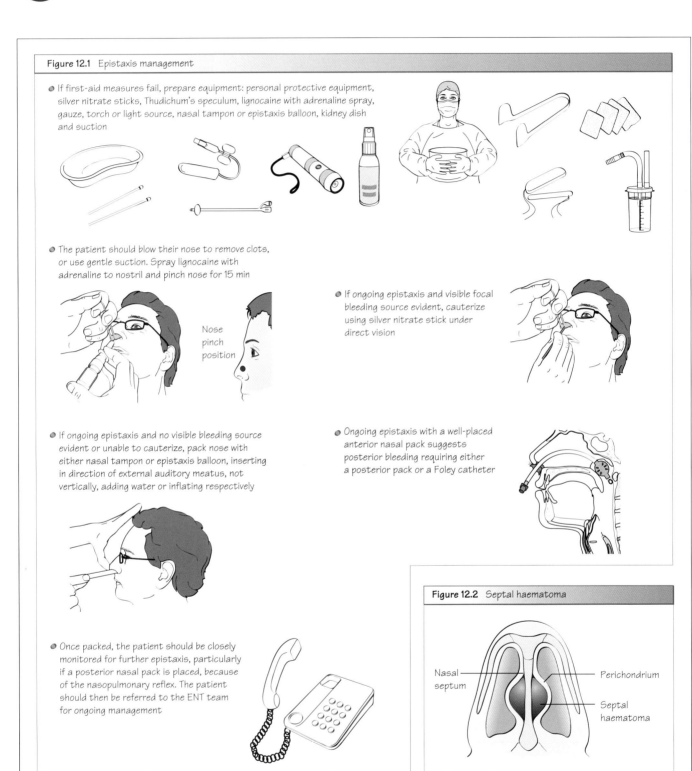

Figure 12.1 Epistaxis management

- If first-aid measures fail, prepare equipment: personal protective equipment, silver nitrate sticks, Thudichum's speculum, lignocaine with adrenaline spray, gauze, torch or light source, nasal tampon or epistaxis balloon, kidney dish and suction

- The patient should blow their nose to remove clots, or use gentle suction. Spray lignocaine with adrenaline to nostril and pinch nose for 15 min

Nose pinch position

- If ongoing epistaxis and visible focal bleeding source evident, cauterize using silver nitrate stick under direct vision

- If ongoing epistaxis and no visible bleeding source evident or unable to cauterize, pack nose with either nasal tampon or epistaxis balloon, inserting in direction of external auditory meatus, not vertically, adding water or inflating respectively

- Ongoing epistaxis with a well-placed anterior nasal pack suggests posterior bleeding requiring either a posterior pack or a Foley catheter

- Once packed, the patient should be closely monitored for further epistaxis, particularly if a posterior nasal pack is placed, because of the nasopulmonary reflex. The patient should then be referred to the ENT team for ongoing management

Figure 12.2 Septal haematoma

Nasal septum

Perichondrium

Septal haematoma

Minor Injury and Minor Illness at a Glance, First Edition. Edited by Francis Morris, Jim Wardrope, and Shammi Ramlakhan.

Approach to the patient

Nasal problems are encountered on a daily basis. The five cardinal symptoms to elicit when approaching the patient presenting with nasal problems are:
- obstruction
- discharge
- pain
- bleeding
- smell disturbance/loss.

Examination of the nose requires:
- good lighting (torch, otoscope, headlight or head mirror);
- Thudichum's speculum if available;
- positioning the patient with head up tilt of 45°.

Examine the external aspect of the nose by inspection and palpation. Anterior rhinoscopy is performed by tilting the tip of the nose upwards and by using a good light and speculum. Check patency of each nostril by asking the patient to blow out through their nose whilst occluding each nostril in turn. Complete the examination by checking the neck and oral cavity.

Specific conditions

Nasal vestibulitis

Nasal vestibulitis is infection of the skin of the nasal vestibule (nasal skin adjacent to each nostril). It is typically caused by pyogenic staphylococcus and commonly results from excessive nose blowing and nose picking. Infection can range from simple folliculitis of the nasal hairs to crusting and cellulitis of the nasal tip which must be treated aggressively to prevent intracranial spread and the risk of developing cavernous sinus thrombosis.

Treatment is with topical and often oral anti-staphylococcal antibiotics. Incision and drainage of furuncles may also be needed.

Rhinitis

Rhinitis is inflammation and irritation of the nasal mucous membranes, presenting with symptoms of rhinorrhoea, nasal congestion, postnasal drip, sneezing or nasal itch.

- *Allergic rhinitis.* This is the most common cause, with common allergens being pollen, dust and dander. Patients often also experience allergic conjunctival symptoms. Treatment involves nasal decongestants, steroid antihistaminic sprays supplemented by an oral antihistamine if required. Patients with persistent severe symptoms often require formal allergy testing and immunology/allergy clinic follow-up.
- *Infective rhinitis.* Caused by *Rhino* and *Corona* viruses, as well as bacteria, typically also resulting in sinusitis.
- *Non-allergic rhinitis.* This is also known as vasomotor rhinitis, and its aetiology remains poorly understood. It is believed to be caused by non-allergic triggers causing nasal vasodilatation and nasal mucosal oedema. Nasal antihistaminic steroid sprays are the mainstay of treatment.

Epistaxis

This can be distressing for patients but is seldom life threatening.

Ninety per cent of bleeding comes from Kiesselbach's plexus on the antero-inferior nasal septum. The remaining 10% is due to posterior epistaxis, typically arising from a posterior branch of the spheno-palatine artery.

First-aid measures include sitting the patient up leaning forwards, loosening tight clothing, encouraging the patient to blow their nose to clear clots and to spit swallowed blood into a bowl. The patient should pinch the nose for up to 30 min. If ice is available this can be applied to the bridge of the nose and the patient, if able, can also suck on an ice cube to encourage vasoconstriction; 4% lignocaine with 1-in-10 000 adrenaline spray can also be administered. Be aware of severe hypertension.

Persistent epistaxis with a visible anterior bleeding source can be chemically cauterized using a silver nitrate stick under direct vision. Both sides of the septum must never be cauterized at the same time, to prevent septal necrosis.

If attempts to control epistaxis with pressure or cauterization fail, the nose should be packed using a nasal tampon or an epistaxis balloon.

Posterior epistaxis is suggested by persistent bleeding despite the adequate placement of an anterior pack and requires the insertion of a commercially available posterior nasal pack or the passage of a Foley catheter.

All patients with a pack should be referred to the ear, nose and throat (ENT) team.

Patients with posterior packs particularly require close monitoring owing to the nasopulmonary reflex, which can commonly cause brady-dysrhythmia and hypoxia.

Foreign body

These should be removed under direct vision using either forceps or suction after first asking the patient to blow out through the affected nostril whilst occluding the other. In children, the 'mother's kiss' is often used, which is a modification of this whereby the parent blows into the child's mouth whilst occluding the unaffected nostril.

Nasal fracture

Nasal fracture is the most common facial fracture, with patients presenting with deformity, tenderness, swelling and expistaxis in some combination. It can result in unfavourable cosmesis if untreated; 80% of fractures occur at the lower one-third to half of the nasal bone.

Radiological imaging should not be performed in the presence of isolated nasal injury because management is dictated by physical examination alone.

Because swelling often accentuates or mimics deformity, patients with suspected nasal fracture should be followed up in around 7–10 days' time by ENT in case closed reduction is required.

> ▶ **Diagnoses not to be missed**
>
> **Septal haematoma**
>
> This is a serious and relatively common complication of nasal trauma resulting in irreversible septal necrosis due to pressure on the septal cartilage from blood in the subperichondrial space. It requires urgent drainage by ENT followed by antibiotics.

13 Facial injury

Figure 13.1 Maxillary fractures

The maxilla often fractures at four points. Fluid in the antrum is an important clue

Fractures:
Inferior orbital rim
Fronto-zygomatic suture

Zygomatic arch

Lateral wall maxillary antrum

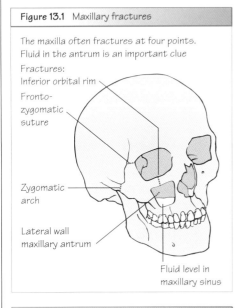

Fluid level in maxillary sinus

Figure 13.2 Blow-out fracture

Note the soft tissue mass below the inferior orbital rim

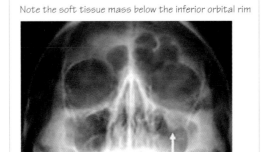

Figure 13.3 Depression of the cheek bones is best noted by looking down from above the head

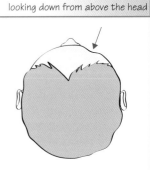

Figure 13.4 Subconjunctival haemorrhage with no posterior limit suggestive of a fracture

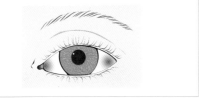

Figure 13.5 Blow-out fracture; pressure inside the orbit increased by squash ball

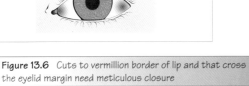

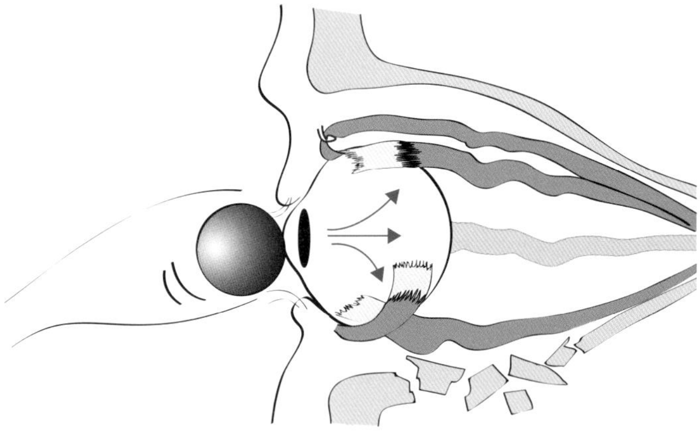

Figure 13.6 Cuts to vermillion border of lip and that cross the eyelid margin need meticulous closure

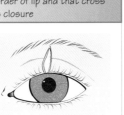

Minor Injury and Minor Illness at a Glance, First Edition. Edited by Francis Morris, Jim Wardrope, and Shammi Ramlakhan.

Approach to the patient

• *History.* The mechanism of injury gives important clues to the diagnosis. What part of the face is involved? Has there been a loss of consciousness? Are the eyes, mouth or ears injured? Is the patient on anticoagulant medication?

• *Examination:*

  ○ *Look* for wounds, bruising, deformity. Check the inside the mouth and the ears.

  ○ *Feel* for exact points of tenderness, especially over the cheek bones, the jaw (especially the temporomandibular joints) and the scalp (scalp wounds are easily overlooked).

  ○ *Move.* Check eye movements, mouth opening and facial movements. Check the nose and ears for bleeding. Check sensation over the cheek (inferior orbital nerve) and over the lower lip (mental nerve). Always assess visual acuity and Glasgow coma score when assessing facial injury.

• *Investigations.* Facial X-rays are often required in blunt injury. If there has been a loss of consciousness a computed tomography (CT) scan may be needed.

Blunt injury

This is the most common mechanism, often due to a fall or a direct blow in sport or during an assault. The common fractures are of the cheek bones (maxilla, including infraorbital floor fracture), jaw (including the mandibular condyle), the zygomatic arch and nasal bones.

Maxillary (cheek bone) fractures

The prominence of the cheek bone is often the first point of contact with a fist or other striking object like a hockey stick. Think of this bone as a four-pointed star (Figure 13.1). Often the bone will break along these four points, the inferior orbital rim, the fronto-zygomatic process, the zygoma and the lateral wall of the maxillary sinus. Exceptions to this are 'blow-out' fractures of the orbit (Figure 13.2) and isolated fractures of the zygomatic process.

Severe trauma can cause complex fractures (le Fort fractures), but these are unlikely to present as minor injuries.

• *Look* for bruising and deformity (best looking down from above; Figure 13.3). Check for subconjunctival haemorrhage, especially where you cannot see the posterior limit (Figure 13.4).

• *Feel.* Check for exact points of tenderness.

• *Move.* Check eye movements, fractures – especially those of the orbital floor can cause diplopia. Check mouth opening and if the teeth meet properly. Always examine the eyes in facial injuries; look for pupillary reaction. Check sensation over the cheek bone and upper lip; the *infraorbital nerve* is often injured in fractures.

Facial X-rays are often needed. Fractures need to be discussed with a facio-maxillary surgeon. If there is diplopia, reduced visual acuity or a significant eye injury, then also discuss with an optholmologist.

A CT scan of the head may be required if there is evidence of associated head injury.

Orbital floor fractures

Pure orbital floor fractures result from impact injury to the globe and upper eyelid. The object is usually large enough not to perforate the globe but small enough not to result in fracture of the orbital rim (Figure 13.5). They are mostly caused by punching injury, secondary to being hit by a squash or tennis ball and road traffic accidents.

• *Examination.* May reveal decreased visual acuity, vertical or oblique diplopia (especially in upward gaze), and decreased sensation in the distribution of the infraorbital nerve. In addition, patients may complain of epistaxis and eyelid swelling following nose blowing. A bony step in the orbital rim and point tenderness may be noted.

• *Investigations.* Facial X rays may show a 'tear drop sign'. Refer to maxillofacial surgeons and also ophthalmologist if associated eye injury is found.

• *Eye injury.* See Chapter 14 for discussion of assessment of eye injuries and less serious injury, such as corneal abrasion.

Jaw injury

Direct blows to the jaw in a fall or assault are the common mechanisms. The patient has pain, local tenderness, is unable to open mouth fully and feels their teeth do not meet normally.

Fractures of the mandibular condyle are caused by transmitted forces and are easily missed.

X-rays include an orthopantogram and oblique views.

Fractures are referred to the maxilla-facial team.

Lacerations

Most wounds to the face are caused by blunt violence. Record the size, position and appearance of the wound. Check for any evidence of fractures or damage the eyes and teeth. Ask if the patient has been knocked out.

ACE wound care (see Chapter 3) is especially important. Cleaning of the wound is especially important as any dirt left in the wound will appear as a tattoo, making the scar much more obvious.

Most wounds can be closed easily. Deep wounds to bone may need to be closed in layers.

Wounds crossing the margins of the eyebrows or the vermillion border of the lip need careful closure (Figure 13.6).

▶ **Diagnoses not to be missed**

- Associated brain injury/traumatic intracranial haemorrhage.
- Associated eye injury.
- Blow-out fractures of the orbit.
- Mandibular condyle injury.
- Injury to facial nerve/parotid duct.

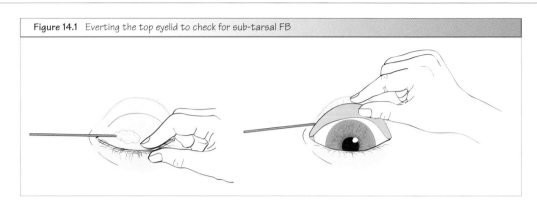

Figure 14.1 Everting the top eyelid to check for sub-tarsal FB

Table 14.1	More serious conditions causing red eye. Do not mis-diagnose these as conjunctivitis. Immediate ophthalmic referral indicated
Anterior uveitis (aka iritis)	Painful unilateral red eye and photophobia. Pupil irregular due to adhesions and poorly reactive. Vision blurry
Keratitis	Painful red eye with photophobia. VA reduced and circumcorneal injection present with a small pupil. Discharge is common
Acute glaucoma	Often onset in dark or stressful situations. Red, painful eye, with nausea and vomiting and haloes. Pupil sluggish and mid-dilated and cornea hazy. The eye feels hard. Refer as an emergency

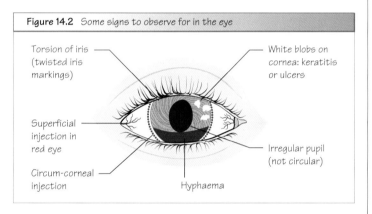

Figure 14.2 Some signs to observe for in the eye

Torsion of iris (twisted iris markings)

White blobs on cornea: keratitis or ulcers

Superficial injection in red eye

Circum-corneal injection

Irregular pupil (not circular)

Hyphaema

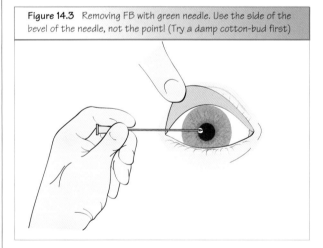

Figure 14.3 Removing FB with green needle. Use the side of the bevel of the needle, not the point! (Try a damp cotton-bud first)

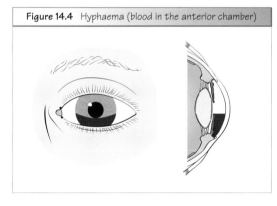

Figure 14.4 Hyphaema (blood in the anterior chamber)

Approach to the patient

Foreign bodies (FBs), corneal abrasions, and conjunctivitis make up the overwhelming majority of problems seen. However, it is important not to miss superficially similar problems which are less common, but more serious (Table 14.1).

The history of the incident is important; for example, FBs are a common complaint, and it should be established whether there is a clear history of injury by an FB or just the sensation of an FB. In addition, a high-speed fragment from shattered metal or a falling piece of rust (with less energy) gives an idea of the potential severity of the injury. Similarly, hammering metal on metal can generate small, high-speed fragments.

Ask about ophthalmic symptoms: loss of vision or of visual field, pain, flashers and floaters. Background history should include general health, as well as ophthalmic history (previous eye treatments, spectacles or contact lenses use).

Examination

All patients should have their visual acuity checked using a Snellen chart (wearing spectacles if used or pinhole if spectacles not present and acuity reduced).

Topical anaesthetic may be required to examine the eye if it is painful. Ensure that any drops are checked – different eye-drops can look very similar and are often stored together. It is not necessary to use an eye pad to provide protection after the use of topical anaesthetic drops.

Examine all the external and anterior structures: lids, lashes, conjunctiva, cornea, anterior chamber and iris/pupils. Unusual iris patterns may be due to penetrating FB or prior surgery. Torsion of the iris or an irregular pupil could be due to iritis or glaucoma. Examine the anterior chambers from the side as well as the front; this may reveal differing degrees of bulge in the chamber, as well as small penetrating FBs.

Pupillary size, symmetry and reaction to light should be checked. If necessary, fluoroscein can be used to demonstrate FBs or abrasions. The eyelids should be everted to check for subtarsal FBs (Figure 14.1) even if another FB has been found embedded in the cornea. Eye movements and visual fields, as well as opthalmoscopy, may be required for unexplained loss of visual acuity.

Further examination

If a slit lamp is available, it can improve the completeness of the examination; however, a safe and adequate examination without a slit lamp is possible. Intra-ocular pressure measurement is rarely available outside of specialist ophthalmic settings.

In cases of acute chemical eye injury, the pH of the eye should be checked with universal pH paper.

Specific conditions: non-traumatic
Conjuctivitis

This presents with a red, watery eye. Occasionally, an FB sensation is present, described as a gritty sensation. Conjunctivitis is often bilateral.

Measured visual acuity should be normal, but a very watery eye may reduce acuity, although this should improve with a pinhole.

An FB or abrasion should be excluded by using flourescein before diagnosing conjunctivitis.

• *Infective conjunctivitis.* May be bacterial or viral. Most cases of conjunctivitis will resolve without treatment within 1–2 weeks. Advise the patient to seek review if the symptoms have not settled in this time or if worsening. If treatment is indicated, topical antibiotic ointment or drops can be used. Conjunctivitis is easily transmissible; therefore, advise hand-washing and avoid sharing towels. If parents are giving the ointment to children they should take particular care to wash hands before and afterwards.

• *Allergic conjunctivitis.* This is nearly always bilateral. Hay-fever (pollen allergy) is a common presenting problem (especially if onset was in the evening after a sunny day). Chemosis (oedema of the conjunctiva) is a classic sign, as is cobble-stone papillae inside the eyelids. Treatment is with topical and/or local antihistamines (available over the counter).

• *Contact lenses.* Conjunctivitis in contact-lens wearers is more likely to be serious or to involve unusual organisms. The patient should stop wearing the lenses, but retain them for cultures. Depending on local policy, immediate or next-day ophthalmic review may be indicated, and/or treatment with ophthalmic antibiotic ointment should be started. White spots on the cornea may be ulcers or infective keratitis – ophthalmic review is always required for these.

Dendritic ulcer

This is not very common and usually presents as a red eye, possibly with an FB sensation. The characteristic spider-like, or branching, ulcer is seen only when stained with fluoroscein or similar. It is caused by the herpes-simplex virus and treatment with antiviral eye-drops and ophthalmic review is indicated.

Subconjunctival haemorrhage

This presents with a bright red demarcated patch on the conjunctiva. The appearance is dramatic, but usually asymptomatic. It results from rupture of a small subconjunctival vessel and blood being visible beneath the conjunctiva.

• *Atraumatic.* Most subconjuctival haemorrhages occur spontaneously. Check the blood pressure for hypertension, and check the INR if the patient is on warfarin. Otherwise, there is no treatment. Reassure the patient – the redness will absorb in about 2 weeks.

• *Ocular injury.* If there is a history of FB, or if the patient was hammering metal, an intra-ocular FB should be excluded.

• *Head injury.* In head injury, subconjunctival haemorrhage is a marker for base of skull fracture. This should be suspected from the history. The haemorrhage will have no definable posterior margin.

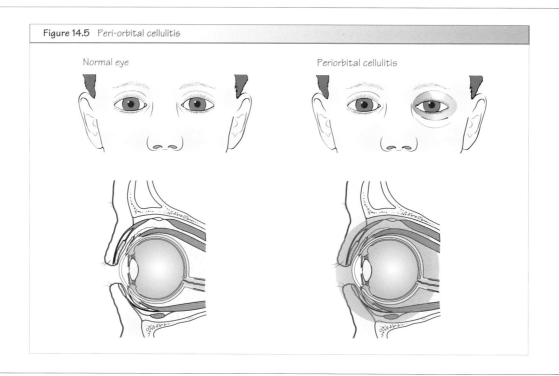

Figure 14.5 Peri-orbital cellulitis

Normal eye   Periorbital cellulitis

► Diagnoses not to be missed

Acute glaucoma (acute-angle closure glaucoma)

Unlike the chronic glaucomas, this presents acutely with a painful red eye. Patients are usually over 60 years old and may also complain of headache, nausea, blurred vision and haloes around lights.

Examination reveals a mid-sized irregular non-reacting pupil.

If suspected, refer urgently to ophthalmology. If you have the facility to check intraocular pressure, this will confirm the diagnosis, but this is not essential.

Peri-orbital cellulitis

Usually presents with painful, unilateral red swollen eyelids (Figure 14.5). The patient is often systemically unwell and may have proptosis, fever, chemosis, reduced vision and limited or painful eye movements.

Remember that not all features will be present. Have a low threshold for considering the diagnosis. Urgent referral and parenteral antibiotics are indicated.

Loss of vision or acute blindness

This can be caused by a variety of conditions; for example, retinal detachment, posterior vitreous detachment, vitreous haemorrhage, central retinal artery occlusion. Some of these have characteristic changes on fundoscopy. A full neurological examination to look for features of a cerebrovascular event with visual field loss (rather than an isolated eye problem) should be performed. Patients should be referred urgently.

More serious causes of red-eye (Table 14.1)

Acute glaucoma and some inflammatory conditions (iritis/uveitis, keratitis) should be considered, especially if there is circumcorneal injection, a fixed or irregular pupil, torsion of the iris, reduced visual acuity, or marked ocular pain and injection. In the presence of these features, urgent ophthalmology referral is recommended.

Giant cell arteritis

This usually occurs in older (over 60) patients with painless visual loss. Headache, scalp tenderness and jaw claudication may be present. This may cause permanent blindness if not treated, and investigation (erythrocyte sedimentation rate), steroid treatment and referral for biopsy are warranted.

Specific conditions: traumatic
Corneal abrasion or foreign body

An FB or FB sensation is one of the most common eye presentations. Patients with conjunctivitis or dendritic ulcer will often give convincing, but misleading, histories of an FB in their eye. Topical anaesthetic can be used to facilitate examination and fluoroscein should help to reveal an FB or corneal abrasion. The eyelids must be everted to check for subtarsal FB.

Superficial FBs should be gently removed with a damp cotton bud. If this fails, embedded FBs can be removed with the edge of the bevel of a needle (Figure 14.3). It is recommended that the needle technique is used in conjunction with a slit lamp to reduce the risks associated with patient movement. If the FB is well embedded and cannot be easily removed, refer to ophthalmology rather than risk further damaging the cornea with repeated attempts at removal.

After removing a metallic FB from the cornea, a rust-ring might be left. These are not usually problematic; however, ophthalmic antibiotic ointment can be prescribed and ophthalmic review arranged in 2–3 days.

A corneal abrasion (including that left by a removed FB) should be treated with ophthalmic antibiotic ointment and review arranged in 2–3 days if symptoms are not settling or if a large abrasion is present.

Chemical injury

Alkaline substances cause more damage than acidic ones, and the pH should be checked with universal indicator/litmus paper for any chemical injury to the eye. Use topical anaesthetic if necessary to allow examination and treatment.

Copious irrigation is the mainstay of treatment, and the eye and conjunctival sacs should be washed with a minimum of 1 L of fluid (normal saline from an intravenous giving set works as well as commercially available irrigation kits).

The pH should be checked again after irrigation. If still abnormal, irrigation should be repeated until the pH is normal (after irrigation, wait a few minutes before rechecking the pH to avoid checking the pH of the irrigation fluid rather than the eye).

After irrigation, examine the eye with fluoroscein for damage and refer to ophthalmology if significant corneal staining/damage seen.

Radiation damage (photokeratitis)

This is commonly caused by welding or observing welding without adequate eye protection ('arc-eye'). Other causes include reflected sunlight (snow blindness). Sun-beds (ultraviolet light) can also cause photokeratitis.

It usually presents with bilateral and very painful tearful eyes after exposure to one of the above conditions. Treatment consists of systemic analgesia, mydriatics and ophthalmic antibiotic ointment. It usually resolves within 36 h.

> ### ▶ Diagnoses not to be missed
>
> #### Penetrating injuries and intraocular foreign body
>
> The signs may be subtle, so suspect this if there is a history of a high energy FB. A small corneal abrasion as well as some distortion to the iris markings or pupil may be the only signs. Carefully examine for a FB. Loss of the red reflex may indicate a vitreous haemorrhage. If suspicious of a penetrating FB, urgent referral to ophthalmology is warranted.
>
> #### Blunt injuries
>
> Small blunt objects (e.g. squash ball, knuckles) can impact directly on the globe, causing bleeding, damage to the iris or lens, or a blowout fracture.
>
> Hyphaema (blood in anterior chamber – Figure 14.4), irregularity of the iris or pupil, altered pupillary reaction or limited eye movement (reduced vertical eye movements indicating a blow-out fracture to the orbital floor) should prompt urgent ophthalmology referral.

15 Mouth and dental

Figure 15.1   Normal adult dentition

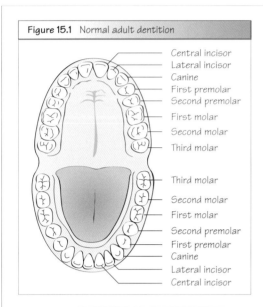

Central incisor
Lateral incisor
Canine
First premolar
Second premolar
First molar
Second molar
Third molar

Third molar
Second molar
First molar
Second premolar
First premolar
Canine
Lateral incisor
Central incisor

Figure 15.2   The oropharynx

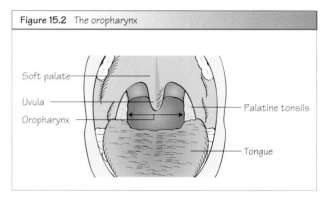

Soft palate
Uvula
Oropharynx
Palatine tonsils
Tongue

Figure 15.3   The lips

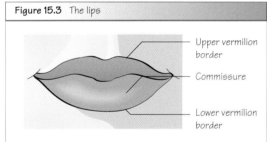

Upper vermilion border
Commissure
Lower vermilion border

Figure 15.4   Dental abscess

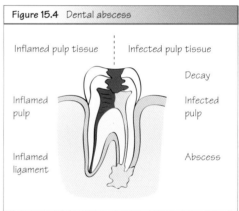

Inflamed pulp tissue
Infected pulp tissue
Decay
Inflamed pulp
Infected pulp
Inflamed ligament
Abscess

Figure 15.5   Swollen salivary glands

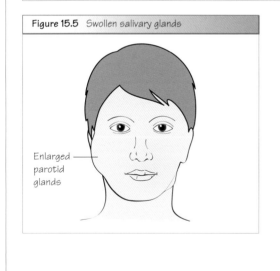

Enlarged parotid glands

Figure 15.6   Ludwig's angina

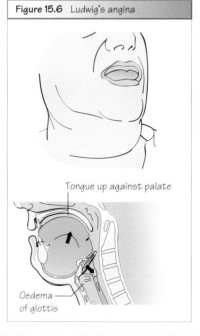

Tongue up against palate
Oedema of glottis

Figure 15.7   Labial frenulum

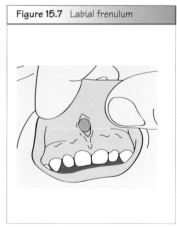

Minor Injury and Minor Illness at a Glance, First Edition. Edited by Francis Morris, Jim Wardrope, and Shammi Ramlakhan.

Approach to the patient

The oropharynx consists of the soft palate and uvula (above), tongue (below), dentition and cheek anterolaterally, tonsils and tonsillar pillars posterolaterally with the pharyngeal wall posteriorly (Figure 15.1).

Dentoalveolar injuries can present in isolation or associated with other injuries, such as mandibular or zygomatic fractures. Take a good history of the mechanism of injury, including the length of time any tooth was avulsed and presence any loose tooth. For ease of examination the patient should be placed in a dental chair or on an examining table at a 45° angle.

Examination should be systematic, beginning with the soft tissues and including the tongue. The base of the tongue is examined for lesions followed by palpation of the submandibular and parotid gland ductal openings. The teeth should be examined next (Figure 15.2). All teeth should be accounted for; if not, a chest X-ray should be performed. Ask the patient to clench their teeth to evaluate their occlusion.

Specific conditions
Dental fractures

The anterior teeth are commonly injured from falls or blows directly to the mouth. Fractures are managed on the basis of the type of fracture and its relation to the pulp. Most patients with dental fractures should be advised to see their dentist. In general, this should be more urgent if the pulp is exposed.

Avulsed teeth

In children with dental avulsions, it is vital not to reimplant the primary teeth because reimplantation of a deciduous tooth can cause harm to the developing permanent tooth.

In adults, reimplantation should be carried out immediately. The goal is to preserve the periodontal ligament. Before implantation, store the tooth in saliva (place tooth in buccal sulcus of patient's mouth), milk or saline. Replace the tooth in the socket after gentle rinsing, and compress the buccal and palatal/lingual alveolar plates. Use a dental anaesthetic if possible, as this can be painful. If the tooth does not seat easily, get the patient to bite on some gauze. The patient should be given oral antibiotics (metronidazole), analgesia and chlorhexidine mouthwash. Tetanus prophylaxis should be administered if necessary, and follow-up arranged with a dentist for splintage.

Lip lacerations

The location and type of injury is important in determining management. The vermilion is the white roll that forms the border between the lip and surrounding skin. This area is the focus of repair because even 1 mm of vermilion misalignment may be noticeable (Figure 15.3). These lacerations should be referred for suturing if the clinician is not confident to do so themselves.

Tongue lacerations

These are mostly due to falls, seizures or other blunt force. Lacerations after a seizure are mostly on the sides of the tongue. Because of the tongue's generous blood supply, most tongue lacerations do not become infected and heal well without repair. Some large, deep or gaping wounds might need repair.

Depending on the skills of the practitioner, minor lacerations can be sutured under local anaesthetic. Otherwise they should be referred to a maxillofacial surgeon.

Dental abscess

These are acute infections characterised by localisation of pus in the structures surrounding the teeth (Figure 15.4). Dental abscesses are mostly caused by mixed anaerobic Gram-negative rods and Gram-positive cocci. The common presentation is of toothache, gum swelling, cheek swelling and if severe, trismus or septicaemia. Analgesics, empirical antibiotics and referral to a dentist are warranted. If the patient is very unwell, there is significant swelling or the infection is spreading, urgent referral to a maxillofacial team is recommended.

Salivary gland problems

Swelling and pain in the salivary glands are often caused by viral infections, of which the most common is mumps (Figure 15.5). This however is becoming rare owing to the MMR vaccination. A stone in the parotid duct may give rise to swelling that gets worse on eating.

Benign and malignant tumours need to be considered in cases of unilateral swelling, particularly if it is relatively painless.

Viral infections need conservative treatment only. For other suspected causes, referral to an ear, nose and throat surgeon is warranted.

▶ Diagnoses not to be missed

Ludwig's angina

This is a rapidly progressive gangrenous cellulitis of the soft tissues of the neck and floor of the mouth due to sepsis in the throat or mouth which migrates to the submandibular space (Figure 15.6). It is more common in diabetic patients.

The most serious and life-threatening complication is airway obstruction due to swelling of the soft tissues and elevation and posterior displacement of the tongue. The patient is ill and toxic with a non-fluctuant swelling below the angle of the jaw. There is oedema of the floor of mouth and around the larynx with elevation and posterior displacement of the tongue. There may be signs of airway obstruction.

Early recognition and hospital admission for empirical broad-spectrum antibiotics, maxillofacial surgical referral for incision and drainage of collections and airway expertise are necessary.

Mouth electrical injuries

These occur commonly in children between the ages of 1 and 2 years when they accidentally bite electrical wires. It causes initial hyperaemia, but swelling of surrounding tissues occurs after a few hours. This can potentially cause airway problems.

These children should be referred urgently to a high-dependency area under a burns specialist and also provided with adequate analgesics.

Labial frenulum injuries

The labial frenulum is the fold of tissue inside the mouth that joins the upper or lower lip to the gums (Figure 15.7).

When present in an abused child, it is frequently associated with multiple injuries; however, a torn frenulum can also occur accidentally if a toddler or young child falls on their face, catches their mouth on low-level furniture or receives an accidental blow to the face. If it remains unexplained in a child under 2 years, assessment should include consideration of other investigations/referral for non-accidental injury as appropriate.

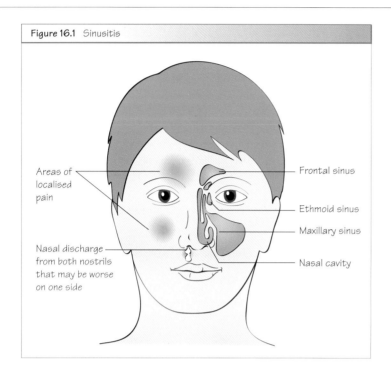

Figure 16.1 Sinusitis

Areas of localised pain

Frontal sinus

Ethmoid sinus

Maxillary sinus

Nasal cavity

Nasal discharge from both nostrils that may be worse on one side

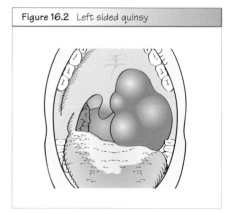

Figure 16.2 Left sided quinsy

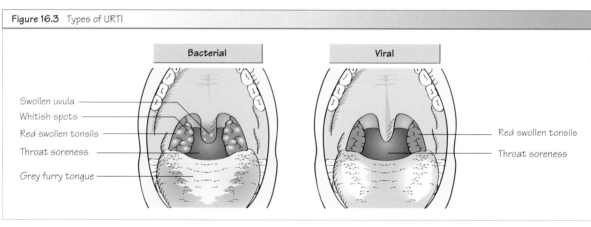

Figure 16.3 Types of URTI

Bacterial

Swollen uvula

Whitish spots

Red swollen tonsils

Throat soreness

Grey furry tongue

Viral

Red swollen tonsils

Throat soreness

Approach to the patient

Upper respiratory infections (URTIs) are normally caused by self-limiting viral illnesses and are one of the most common reasons patients seek medical advice. Viral URTIs, although normally mild, can cause significant concern to patients, with anxiety, inappropriate treatments and missed work. In patients with concomitant chronic diseases, extreme age or frailty a URTI can cause significant social and medical morbidity. Concerns about transmission to others may also be important in the recovery. Always check vital signs, look for signs of dehydration and assess if the patient looks ill. Examine the upper and lower respiratory tract to exclude lower respiratory infection. Antibiotics will not speed or aid the recovery of a viral infection or prevent sequelae, including bacterial lower respiratory tract infection, and so should be avoided in uncomplicated URTI as they can have side effects and promote antibiotic resistance in the population.

Minor Injury and Minor Illness at a Glance, First Edition. Edited by Francis Morris, Jim Wardrope, and Shammi Ramlakhan.

Specific conditions
Viral cold

Most URTIs are caused by the common cold virus. Symptoms of coryza (cough and nasal mucus), fever (usually <38°C), myalgia and tiredness will normally last 1–2 weeks, but duration is normally unimportant. Advise over the counter analgesia, decongestant and cough suppressing therapy. If there is a productive cough then a lower respiratory tract bacterial infection should be suspected. Post-viral cough can occur, but if prolonged then carcinoma of bronchus may need to be excluded.

Influenza

Caused by the influenza virus and normally occurring in the context of seasonal flu outbreak or pandemic infection (e.g. 2009 H1N1 swine flu pandemic). Influenza is normally a worse and longer illness than that caused by the common cold virus, with more lethargy, malaise and higher fevers. Guidance from local and national virology departments should be followed with regard to investigation and treatment. At-risk patients with comorbidities, who are pregnant or immunosupressed may need swabs for diagnosis and treatment with antiviral drugs such as oseltamivir or Oseltamivir. Prophylactic antiviral drugs can be used in epidemics under the guidance of public health departments to prevent spread.

Most people fully recover within 2 weeks with no treatment, and some strains can give a mild illness only.

Tonsilitis

Many cases are caused by viruses, but bacterial infections, particularly group A beta haemolytic streptococcus, are relatively common. Streptococcal tonsillitis can cause significant complications, such as glomerulonephritis, rheumatic fever, peritonsillar abscess (quinsy) and Kawasaki disease. While these complications are rare, antibiotics are advised if streptococcal infection is suspected.

Symptoms usually consist of soreness and swelling of the tonsils, painful swallowing, lymphadenopathy, with fever and sometimes a rash (scarlet fever). Visual examination cannot distinguish consistently between viral and bacterial tonsillitis. But for mild viral infections supportive treatment is sufficient.

Tests are usually not necessary, though the specific organism can be identified by taking a throat swab in cases where the diagnosis is uncertain or in initial treatment failure. Amoxicilin is normally avoided in case the tonsillitis is caused by Epstein–Barr virus (glandular fever), where a florid rash can be caused by the reaction of virus and drug.

Sinusitis

Infection of the sinuses next to the nasal passages can cause fever, nasal discharge, facial/dental pain and congestion. It is usually viral or bacterial and the location of the pain depends on which sinus is affected.

Self-treatment with a short course of nasal or oral decongestants, regular steam inhalation to relieve congestion and Eustachian tube dysfunction and analgesia are normally enough. If prolonged or severe then antibiotics can be needed. Long-lasting sinusitis more than 2 months is chronic sinusitis and usually needs referral to an otolaryngologist to consider further imaging or treatment. Surgical drainage can be performed by a specialist for these cases.

Abscess, ocular, meningeal or cerebral involvement can occur in rare circumstances, so any neurological or visual defects should be investigated urgently.

Diagnoses not to be missed
Quinsy

Peritonsillar abscess (quinsy) appears as a large swelling forming outside the tonsil's capsule on one tonsil as a complication of bacterial tonsillitis. It presents with unremitting fever, pooling of saliva and dehydration (due to severe pain on swallowing and dysphagia). Systemic antibiotic treatment and incision and drainage are the necessary treatments, most commonly done by an otolaryngologist. Tonsillectomy is commonly carried out at a later date to prevent further episodes. Failure to recognise and treat quinsy can lead to severe dehydration and septicaemia.

Lower respiratory tract disease

See Chapter 17.

Head and neck malignancy

Malignancy in the nose/sinuses or pharynx is very uncommon. It can present late with no early symptoms. Suspect malignancy in patients with weight loss, prolonged night sweats, lymphadenopathy, neurological or visual problems. In the nasal/sinus area, it should be considered if there is blood/unilateral nasal obstruction in association with the URTI symptoms, swelling of the face, ocular symptoms or headaches. In the pharyngeal area it may cause dysphagia, haemoptysis, hoarseness or neck swelling. Computed tomography or magnetic resonance imaging with referral to an otolaryngologist will be needed if suspected.

Septicaemia

Many severe systemic illnesses can in early stages be confused with cold or flu symptoms; for example, meningococcaemia or pneumonia. Unremitting/high fever, bruising, joint pains, non-blanching rash, rigors, chest pain, seizure, diminished conscious level, confusion, dehydration or shock should all be symptoms of concern that may suggest sepsis. Resuscitation and urgent antimicrobial treatment should be urgently commenced and the patient referred to hospital.

Epiglotitis

Although very rare since routine immunisation with *Haemophilus influenzae* B (HiB) vaccine, this condition still occurs, especially in adults who have not been immunised. The condition can be caused by other bacteria (*Streptococcus*, *Staphylococcus* and *Moraxella catarrhalis*). Because of HiB vaccine the incidence of epiglottitis is proportionally increasing in adults compared with children. It can cause stridor and respiratory distress, leading to airway obstruction and death. Early treatment with parenteral antibiotics and expert airway management is essential. Vigorous attempts to examine the pharynx should be avoided as this may cause a life-threatening laryngopharyngeal spasm leading to a rapid worsening of the patient's condition.

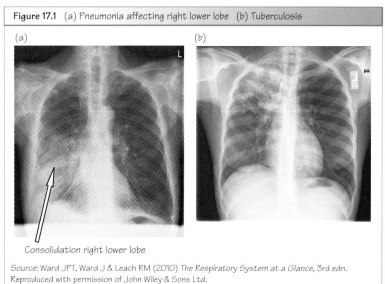

Figure 17.1 (a) Pneumonia affecting right lower lobe (b) Tuberculosis

(a)

(b)

Consolidation right lower lobe

Source: Ward JPT, Ward J & Leach RM (2010) *The Respiratory System at a Glance*, 3rd edn. Reproduced with permission of John Wiley & Sons Ltd.

Table 17.1 CRB-65 score

Score 1 point for each of:
• Confusion (mental test score <8 or new disorientation)
• Respiratory rate >30/min
• Blood pressure (SBP<90 mmHg or DBP <60 mmHg)
• Age >65 years

CRB-65 score (Associated mortality)	0 (1.2%)	1 or 2 (5–12%)	3 or 4 (33–48%)
	Likely suitable for home treatment	Consider hospital referral	Urgent hospital admission

Source: Ward JPT, Ward J & Leach RM (2010)
The Respiratory System at a Glance, 3rd edn.
Reproduced with permission of John Wiley & Sons Ltd

Table 17.2 Causes and specific features of community-acquired pneumonia

Pathogen	% cases	Specific features
Streptococcus pneumoniae	60–75	Commonest in winter months. Lobar involvement >> bronchopneumonic pattern. Rapid onset, high fever, herpes labialis, vomiting. Mortality 5–10%
Mycoplasma pneumoniae	5–18	Mainly in autumn. Epidemics every 3–4 years. Complications (20%): myocarditis, meningo-encephalitis, rash, haemolytic anaemia (cold haemagglutinin)
Haemophilus influenzae	4–5	Bronchopneumonia. Usually underlying lung disease
Legionella	2–5	Commonest in autumn in previously healthy individuals, from contaminated air conditioning. Key features: confusion, hepatitis, renal impairment, ↓Na+
Chlamydia psittaci	2	From infected birds. Protracted illness. 50% hepato-splenomegaly
Staphylococcus aureus	1–5	During influenza A epidemics. Rapid progression and high mortality (30%). Cavitation in 50%, pleural effusion/empyema in 15%, pneumothorax
Gram-negative pneumonia	10	Underlying illness, often chronic. Increased chance in nosocomial infections. Often severe pneumonia, with septic shock. Klebsiella, Pseudomonas, E. coli
Influenza	5–8	Preceding myalgia + severe prostration. Epidemic
Other	2–8	

Source: Davey P (ed.) (2010) *Medicine at a Glance*, 3rd edn. Reproduced with permission of John Wiley & Sons Ltd

Table 17.3 Risk factors for pneumonia

- Age: >65, <5 years old
- Chronic disease (e.g. renal and lung)
- Diabetes mellitus
- Immunosuppression (e.g. drugs and HIV)
- Alcohol dependency
- Aspiration (e.g. epilepsy)
- Recent viral illness (e.g. influenza)
- Malnutrition
- Mechanical ventilation
- Postoperative (e.g. obesity and smoking)
- Environmental (e.g. psittacosis)
- Occupational (e.g. Q fever)
- Travel abroad (e.g. paragonimiasis)
- Air conditioning (e.g. Legionella)

Approach to patient

Infections in the lower airways are common and the clinical presentation may vary from a well patient with a cough, to those with severe sepsis. Many patients do not require hospital admission and can be managed with oral antibiotics. A thorough assessment is important in all cases, as many of the symptoms are nonspecific and could be related to other serious conditions. Particular care needs to be taken to look for the signs of sepsis or malignancy, especially in the elderly or smokers.

Specific conditions
Acute bronchitis

The presence of an acute cough or acute bronchitis can last up to 3 weeks. Patients may also complain of fever, headache, cold symptoms and myalgia. It is a self-limiting condition associated with a viral infection. Patients should be advised to rest and drink plenty of fluids. They should also be told to stop smoking as bronchitis, chest infections and chronic obstructive pulmonary disease (COPD) are all associated with smoking. Regular paracetamol should also be advised.

Minor Injury and Minor Illness at a Glance, First Edition. Edited by Francis Morris, Jim Wardrope, and Shammi Ramlakhan.

Chest infections

These patients also complain of cough. The absence of any abnormal signs on examination (pulse, respiratory rate, temperature and no focal chest signs on examination) makes the diagnosis of radiologically defined pneumonia unlikely. Most will have a non-pneumonic lower respiratory tract infection (LRTI).

Antibiotics are of no benefit in non-pneumonic LRTIs, which are associated with viral infection. Unnecessary antibiotic prescribing can cause side effects and can lead to the development of resistant bacteria, potentially making further infections more difficult to treat.

Pneumonia

Common symptoms are of fever, cough and sputum production. The patient may also complain of dyspnoea, pleuritic chest pain, rigors, haemoptysis and myalgia. Elderly patients may present with malaise, anorexia, myalgia or an episode of collapse.

Signs include tachypnoea, pyrexia, crepitations and/or bronchial breathing on auscultation and dullness to percussion.

The diagnosis is based on having signs and symptoms of LRTI and new consolidation on chest X-ray (CXR).

Some patients present with these symptoms but are only mildly unwell and may be safely managed with appropriate antibiotics, simple analgesia and advice to drink plenty and not to smoke. Follow-up should be arranged to ensure resolution. A repeat CXR at 6 weeks is recommended.

Patients most at risk from pneumonia are the immunocompromised (those with diabetes, cystic fibrosis, HIV, on steroids) and those with any chronic health condition.

The CRB-65 (Table 17.1) score is used to help assess severity of illness; however, always consider individual patient circumstances and home support. Mortality from community-acquired pneumonia is less than 1% in those well enough to be managed at home.

The CRB-65 score does not include hypoxia. If any patient is significantly more hypoxic than normal then they are likely to need admission to hospital.

Choice of antibiotics depends on the likely organism. Most commonly this will be *Streptococcus pneumoniae* (33%), so amoxicillin or clarithromycin (if penicillin allergic) for 5 days is a good choice.

Atypical pathogens are influenza A virus, *Mycoplasma pneumoniae*, *Haemophilus influenzae*, *Chlamydophila psittaci*, *Legionella pneumophila*, *Coxiella burnetti* and *Staphylococcus aureus* (Table 17.2). Chest signs can be minimal and there is often discordance between the chest signs and the illness of the patient. The CXR can appear florid and thus raises the suspicion of an atypical pathogen. There may be signs in other systems due to complications.

There is no evidence that routinely giving antibiotics against the atypicals leads to better outcomes in non-severe illness. Macrolides are effective in all three of the most common atypicals, although there is growing concern about the development of resistance.

Exacerbations of chronic obstructive pulmonary disease

Patients with COPD often attend with increasing dyspnoea, cough, sputum production and purulence, with or without symptoms of upper respiratory infection. In COPD, antibiotics should only be used when there is a history of more purulent sputum, and only purulent sputum should be sent for culture. There is good evidence that green purulent sputum is a good indicator of high bacterial load and that patients without purulence will improve without antibiotics. Doxycyline is recommended. Nebulisers and/or increased use of inhalers may also be necessary.

Patients with new consolidation on a CXR should be treated as a community-acquired pneumonia.

Other conditions, such as heart failure, pulmonary embolus and pneumothorax, may have similar presentations, so it is essential to perform a thorough assessment.

Aspiration pneumonia

This is a chemical pneumonitis that commonly occurs after aspiration. It is most common in patients who have swallowing difficulties (e.g. post stroke, degenerative neurological conditions). Bacterial pneumonia may follow after 2–5 days in 25–50% of cases but is not prevented by early prophylactic antibiotics. Antibiotics should only be considered if aspiration pneumonitis fails to resolve by 48 h after aspiration, the sputum becomes purulent or other features consistent with pneumonia develop. These patients clearly need hospital admission and intravenous antibiotics.

Asthma

A LRTI can trigger an acute attack of asthma. These are often viral and may not need antibiotics. It is vital to check the patient's peak flow and respiratory rate in order to assess how unwell they are. The acute asthma guidelines should then be followed. All asthmatics who present with a peak expiratory flow rate <50% should have steroids (40–50 mg oral prednisolone) and be given nebulised salbutamol initially. A CXR is only indicated in those patients who have life-threatening asthma, a suspected pneumothorax, suspected consolidation, those who are failing to respond to treatment adequately and those who need invasive ventilation.

Tuberculosis

In the UK the number of tuberculosis (TB) cases is again rising. Alcoholics, HIV-positive individuals, some recent immigrants and healthcare workers are at increased risk. Symptoms are of a chronic or persistent cough and sputum production. If the disease is at an advanced stage the sputum will contain blood. Patients may also complain of fatigue, reduced appetite, weight loss, fever and night sweats.

> ### ▶ Diagnoses not to be missed
>
> - If a cough persists for more than 3–4 weeks there could be an underlying malignancy or TB. Patients who complain of this should have a thorough examination and a CXR.
> - If becomes short of breath, has a severe wheeze, severe headache or severe chest pain. If the patient appears very unwell they need a full and thorough assessment as they could have severe pneumonia, severe acute asthma, an atypical pneumonia, pulmonary embolus or myocardial infarction.
> - If has haemoptysis they could have pneumonia; other causes include pulmonary embolus (see Chapter 18), malignancy or TB.
> - If becomes confused or drowsy, they may well be hypoxic. Confusion, particularly in the elderly patient, can be one of the few signs that they have pneumonia.

Table 18.1 Indications for X-ray in chest trauma

Significant mechanism of injury
Shortness of breath
Hypoxia/high respiratory rate
Suspected haemothorax/pneumothorax
Elderly patients
Significant pre-existing chest problems

Table 18.2 Non traumatic chest pain causes

Heart	Lungs	Mediastinum	Abdomen	Chest Wall
Myocardial ischaemia	Pneumonia	Dissecting aortic aneurism	Gastric ulcer	Musculo-skeletal
Myocardial infarction	Pneumothorax	Oesophageal problems	Gallstones	Costo chondritis
Pericarditis	Pulmonary embolus		Pancreatitis	Herpes zoster

Table 18.3 Major categories of chest pain

Musculoskeletal
Myocardial ischaemia – often dull, heavy or pressing, radiating to arm/neck/jaw
Pleuritic – often sharp, worse on deep breathing
Tearing – dissecting aortic aneurysm
Atypical – none of above

Table 18.4 Patients with atypical chest pain who require further investigation

Severe pain
Unwell
Elderly
Risk factors for acute coronary syndrome
Risk factors for pulmonary embolism
Abnormal vital signs
Abnormal examination
Persistent/recurring symptoms

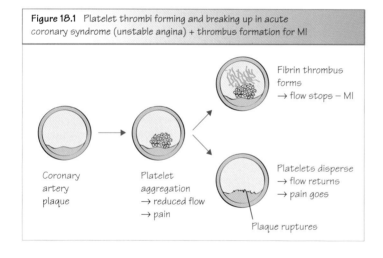

Figure 18.1 Platelet thrombi forming and breaking up in acute coronary syndrome (unstable angina) + thrombus formation for MI

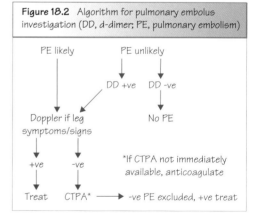

Figure 18.2 Algorithm for pulmonary embolus investigation (DD, d-dimer; PE, pulmonary embolism)

Minor chest injury

- **History.** The common mechanisms are falls, seat belt injury and direct blows in sport or in an assault. Older patients are more likely to have complications.
- **Examination.** Always check vital signs. *Look* for any bruising, *feel* for the exact points of tenderness, crepitus or 'crackling' (subcutaneous emphysema). In road traffic accidents and in the elderly check the sternum and spine. Ask the patient to take a deep breath (*move*). Percuss and listen for breath sounds. Examine the abdomen for any signs of tenderness.

- **Investigations.** Most patients will *not* need a chest X-ray. In seat belt injuries, an X-ray of the sternum may be needed. Table 18.1 lists the indications for X-ray.
- **Plan.** Tell the patient they have bruised or cracked a rib. This is very painful. Give good analgesia. Tell the patient to take deep breaths regularly, holding the painful area. They should do the same when they cough or laugh. They should return if they become unwell or if the pain is uncontrolled.

Minor Injury and Minor Illness at a Glance, First Edition. Edited by Francis Morris, Jim Wardrope, and Shammi Ramlakhan.

Fractured sternum

Usually occurs from impact on the steering wheel or from the seatbelt. There is severe anterior chest wall pain with localised tenderness over the sternum. Perform an electrocardiogram (ECG) as there could be a cardiac contusion. If there are any ECG changes then cardiac enzymes should be measured and the patient admitted. The injury can also be associated with great vessel injury and spinal injury.

Treatment is analgesia. Patients with an isolated sternal fracture, a normal ECG, no other major injuries and no significant pre-existing medical problems can be discharged.

Non-traumatic chest pain

See Table 18.2 for diagnoses not to be missed.

Risk assessment is based on a good history. Examination is often normal, even in serious illness. Investigations are often required.
• *History.* Take a full 'SOCRATES' history of the pain. Severe chest pain of sudden onset needs further investigation. There are four major types of chest pain (see Table 18.3). Past history is especially important.
• *Examination.* Check the vital signs. Perform a general examination – does the patient look unwell? Examine the cardiovascular and respiratory systems. Examine the abdomen.
• *Investigation.* This will depend entirely on the history and examination. Very often an ECG is indicated. It is difficult to exclude serious pathology without blood test and a chest X-ray.

Musculoskeletal pain is very common, worse with specific movements and the chest wall may be tender. It is a common diagnosis usually made once more serious conditions have been excluded.

Ischaemic chest pain

The pain is usually central, often a dull ache, often with radiation to the arms or jaw. Angina is common. The pain usually lasts for less than 15 min. Patients with stable angina will often be able to manage their own symptoms. If their angina is lasting longer, is not responding to usual management or coming on much more frequently then they will need investigation.

Acute coronary syndrome includes unstable angina, non-ST-elevation myocardial infarction (MI) and ST-elevation MI and is caused by rupture of a coronary artery plaque.
• *History.* Symptoms can come and go, as platelet thrombus form and disperse (Figure 18.1). Cardiac risk factors include smoking, diabetes, hypercholesterolaemia, family history, hypertension, previous ischaemic heart disease.
• *Examination.* This is often normal.
• *Investigations.* Patients with new-onset significant chest pain need investigation with ECG, cardiac enzymes and a chest X-ray.
• *Plan.* Patients with sudden onset, severe, central, crushing chest pain and new ECG changes need to be referred to a cardiologist immediately.

Atypical presentations are common and include indigestion-type pain, pain with musculoskeletal features or no pain (especially in diabetics and the elderly) who may have left ventricular failure, collapse or confusion.

Pleuritic chest pain

The pain is worse on deep breathing. Important diagnoses are are given in Table 2. Pneumonia, pulmonary embolism and pneumothorax are common serious conditions.
• *History.* A full 'OPQSRT' history of the pain is needed. Other symptoms, such as cough, fever, sputum production, leg symptoms and previous history should be asked. Check if pregnant.
• *Examination.* Vital signs and general examination give important clues. Examine the chest, abdomen and legs.
• *Investigation.* This will depend on the findings on history and examination. If the patient is unwell then chest X-ray is advisable. If there is a significant possibility of pulmonary embolism then further tests, such as d-dimer or computed tomography pulmonary angiography (CTPA), will be needed.

Pulmonary embolism

Physical signs can be very difficult to detect in small pulmonary emboli. Look for any signs of deep vein thrombosis in the legs. A pre-test probability should be calculated (refer to your hospital guidelines). Figure 18.2 outlines a treatment algorithm for suspected pulmonary embolus.

Pneumonia

Pain, fever, green sputum would suggest pneumonia. Young fit patients who look well may be treated in the community. Patients who are unwell, older or have pre-existing chest disease may need hospital assessment (see Chapter 17).

Spontaneous pneumothorax

Occurs most commonly in thin young men and in those with pre-existing chest disease. Diagnosis is by chest X-ray.

Aortic dissection

Patients with sudden-onset severe tearing pain in the anterior or posterior chest need immediate referral to hospital. The majority of patients have a hypertension. It can also follow recent cardiac surgery or angioplasty. It is also associated with Marfan's, Ehlers–Danlos and a bicuspid aortic valve. Mortality is around 30%.

Patient with a typical history will need computed tomography angiography.

> ### ◤ Diagnoses not to be missed
>
> Atypical chest pain can be real diagnostic challenge. The pain is often non-specific and the cause not found. Oesphageal pain, pain radiating from the abdomen, musculoskeletal chest wall pain may present in this way. However, acute coronary syndrome, pulmonary embolism, pneumonia and aortic dissection can also all present atypically.
>
> Table 18.4 lists features that would indicate investigation is needed.

19 Abdominal pain

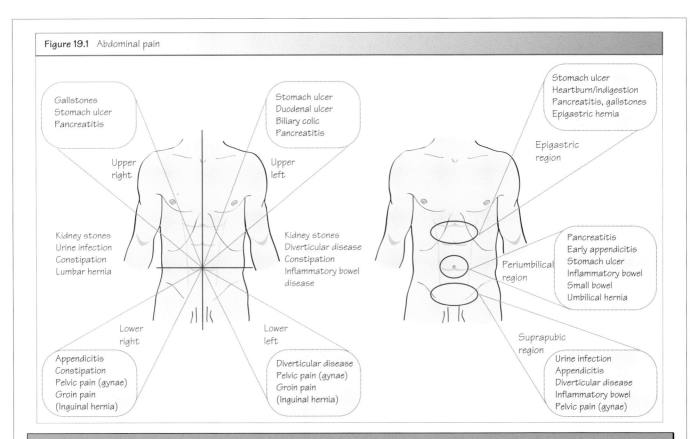

Figure 19.1 Abdominal pain

Gallstones
Stomach ulcer
Pancreatitis

Stomach ulcer
Duodenal ulcer
Biliary colic
Pancreatitis

Upper right

Upper left

Kidney stones
Urine infection
Constipation
Lumbar hernia

Kidney stones
Diverticular disease
Constipation
Inflammatory bowel disease

Lower right

Lower left

Appendicitis
Constipation
Pelvic pain (gynae)
Groin pain
(Inguinal hernia)

Diverticular disease
Pelvic pain (gynae)
Groin pain
(Inguinal hernia)

Stomach ulcer
Heartburn/indigestion
Pancreatitis, gallstones
Epigastric hernia

Epigastric region

Periumbilical region

Pancreatitis
Early appendicitis
Stomach ulcer
Inflammatory bowel
Small bowel
Umbilical hernia

Suprapubic region

Urine infection
Appendicitis
Diverticular disease
Inflammatory bowel
Pelvic pain (gynae)

Table 19.1 Abdominal pain

	Typical symptoms	Typical signs	Atypical symptoms/signs
Ulcer disease	Epigastic pain, nausea	Usually well with soft abdomen (unless perforated)	If perforated – unwell, rigid abdomen
Appendicitis	Umbilical pain that moves to the right iliac fossa, nausea	Unwell, foetor, tender right iliac fossa guarding	In pelvic appendix may have some urinary symptoms and flank pain if retrocaecal
Cholecystitis /biliary colic	Right upper quadrant pain, radiating to back, vomiting, loss of appetite	Unwell, right upper quadrant tenderness	May present with back pain, epigastric pain
Pancreatitis	Severe upper/generalised pain, vomiting	Very unwell, may be shocked, very tender, rigid abdomen	May present with chest pain
Aortic aneurysm	Severe, sudden onset abdominal or back pain	Very unwell, shocked, tender pulsatile mass	May present solely with back pain. If the bleed is small, shock may be absent
Obstruction	Colicky pain, vomiting, not passing flatus	Unwell, may have distension. Check hernial orifices carefully	Vomiting may be late in large bowel obstruction
Mesenteric ischaemia	Older patient or atrial fibrillation. Often non specific symptoms	Unwell, shocked, abdomen difficult to examine but often no clear signs	
Diverticular disease	Older patient, lower abdominal pain	Well and soft abdomen unless abscess or perforated	
Myocardial infarction/ pnuemonia	Upper abdominal pain, may be vomiting. sweating	No signs in abdomen	
Diabetic ketoacidosis/ septicaemia	Generalised abdominal pain	Very unwell, dry, abdomen soft	
Pelvic/ urinary problems	See Chapters 20 and 22		

Minor Injury and Minor Illness at a Glance, First Edition. Edited by Francis Morris, Jim Wardrope, and Shammi Ramlakhan.

Approach to the patient

There are many causes of abdominal pain in adults (Table 19.1). Some of these can lead to cardiovascular instability. Initial assessment and, if required, resuscitation are important.

Once the patient is stabilised, a good history is key to the diagnosis (see SOCRATES, Chapter 1, Figure 1.2). Three aspects of the history are particularly important:
- site of the pain (and if the site changes);
- character of the pain;
- associated symptoms (particularly gastrointestinal, gynaecological and genitourinary symptoms).

Following a focused history, physical examination can confirm the suspected diagnosis. General examination may reveal signs of dehydration, fever, anaemia or jaundice. Check for foetor on the breath. Carefully palpate the abdomen to locate the exact site of tenderness, any protective muscle spasm (guarding) and percussion tenderness (Figure 19.1). Consider the need for examination of the rectum, vagina, hernia orifices and external genitalia in the male.

Urinalysis and urinary pregnancy testing are essential.

Specific causes of abdominal pain

Common causes of abdominal pain can be categorised by site of pain and system affected. A few extra-abdominal causes of abdominal pain should also be considered in all adults, such as myocardial infarction, pneumonia and diabetic ketoacidosis.

Upper abdominal pain

Gastrointestinal causes
- *Peptic ulcer disease.* Usually presents with a sudden onset of epigastric pain with vomiting. The patient has epigastric tenderness. A history of nonsteroidal anti-inflammatory drug or alcohol use may be elicited. Examination may reveal epigastric tenderness; guarding or rebound tenderness suggests perforation.
- *Acute cholecystitis.* Often affects obese females, and the patient may have a past history of similar pain. The pain is colicky in nature and sited in the right upper quadrant. Examination may elicit a positive Murphy's sign (the patient experiences pain and catches their breath on breathing deeply while the examining hand presses on the right upper quadrant).
- *Acute pancreatitis.* Usually seen in patients with gallstones or in alcoholics. Patients present with severe epigastric pain, prostration and vomiting. Patients may be unstable and require aggressive resuscitation. An elevated serum lipase is diagnostic.

Genitourinary causes
- *Ureteric colic.* Usually presents in young adult men. Pain is colicky and radiates from loin to groin. Haematuria is almost always present. A bedside ultrasound may aid in diagnosis and demonstrate hydronephrosis. Patients with ureteric colic, hydronephrosis and fever require urgent urological consultation.

Other causes
- *Aortic aneurysm.* Presents with abdominal pain radiating through to the back, but may mimic any other cause of abdominal pain. This condition must be suspected in all patients over 55 years presenting with abdominal pain. Examination may reveal a tender pulsatile aorta. Urgent vascular surgical consultation is required.
- *Diabetic ketoacidosis.* May present with central abdominal pain and vomiting, in the absence of specific abdominal pathology. Always check the blood glucose in all patients presenting with nonspecific abdominal pain, dehydration and prostration. Patients with diabetic ketoacidosis and abdominal pain should be investigated for an abdominal pathology predisposing to diabetic ketoacidosis (such as pyelonephritis).
- *Acute myocardial infarction.* May present as upper abdominal pain, nausea and cold sweats. All adult patients presenting with undiagnosed upper abdominal pain should have a 12-lead electrocardiogram as part of their initial assessment.

Lower abdominal pain

Gastrointestinal causes
- *Acute appendicitis.* Presents with central abdominal pain that migrates eventually to the right lower quadrant. Patients are usually anorexic and nauseous. Appendicitis may mimic most other causes of lower abdominal pain. Urinary symptoms can be present. Most patients are diagnosed on clinical grounds, but in doubtful cases ultrasound can be useful.
- *Acute diverticulitis.* Is a condition of the elderly. Patients present with left lower quadrant pain and fever. On examination of the abdomen there is tenderness in the left lower quadrant, often with guarding and rebound tenderness. Patients are often dehydrated and may be septic and haemodynamically unstable.
- *Ischaemic colitis.* Is also a condition of the elderly. It should be considered in any elderly patient presenting with severe abdominal pain, but minimal signs on physical examination.

Genitourinary causes
- *Urinary tract infection.* Severe urinary tract infection may cause lower abdominal pain, but if pain is severe there will be other urinary symptoms. Urinary tract infections are probably overdiagnosed in patients with abdominal pain.
- *Testicular torsion.* May present as acute, severe abdominal pain in adolescents or young men. The pain is often associated with prostration and vomiting. See Chapter 21.

All females of child-bearing age presenting with abdominal pain must have a urinary pregnancy test as part of their initial work-up. See Chapter 22.

 Diagnoses not to be missed

Certain presentations of abdominal pain present a diagnostic challenge for the clinician, and some general rules of caution must be applied in these situations.

Abdominal pain in the elderly

Elderly patients with abdominal pain can be difficult to diagnose and manage. There are several reasons for this:
- symptoms and signs are often nonspecific in this age group;
- patients often appear less ill than they actually are;
- several life-threatening conditions are more common in the elderly;
- elderly patients have less physiological reserve and are likely to decompensate rapidly and without warning.

In any elderly patients presenting with abdominal pain, the following diagnoses should always be considered:
- abdominal aortic aneurysm;
- ischaemic colitis;
- myocardial infarction.

However, it should be remembered that elderly patients can also present with almost all of the conditions seen in younger adults.

Figure 20.1 Using urine dipstick to diagnose urinary tact infections (UTI)

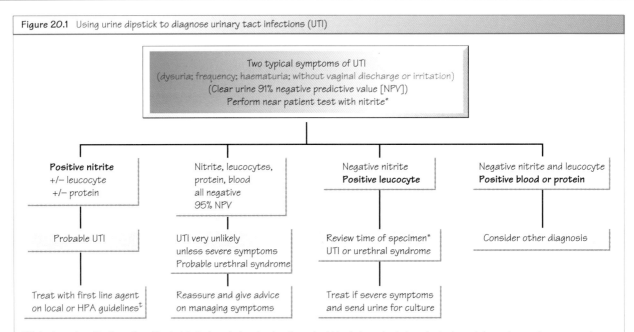

Two typical symptoms of UTI
(dysuria; frequency; haematuria; without vaginal discharge or irritation)
(Clear urine 91% negative predictive value [NPV])
Perform near patient test with nitrite*

Positive nitrite
+/− leucocyte
+/− protein

Nitrite, leucocytes,
protein, blood
all negative
95% NPV

Negative nitrite
Positive leucocyte

Negative nitrite and leucocyte
Positive blood or protein

Probable UTI

UTI very unlikely
unless severe symptoms
Probable urethral syndrome

Review time of specimen*
UTI or urethral syndrome

Consider other diagnosis

Treat with first line agent
on local or HPA guidelines[t]

Reassure and give advice
on managing symptoms

Treat if severe symptoms
and send urine for culture

*Nitrite is produced by the action of bacterial nitrate reductase in urine. As contact time between bacteria and urine is needed, morning specimens are most reliable. Leucocyte esterase detects intact and lysed leucocytes produced in inflammation. Haematuria and proteinuria occur in UTI but are also present in other conditions. When reading test **WAIT** for the time recommended by manufacturer.
t = http://www.hpa.org.uk/infections/topics_az/antimicrobial_resistance/guidance.htm
 Urethral syndrome: a syndrome characterised by symptoms identical to urinary tract infection (e.g. frequency, suprapubic pain, dysuria) but in which no microbes are found to colonise the urinary tract. Other conditions affecting the uro-gynaecological tract need to be ruled out; in many the cause remains unclear
From Health Protection Agency www.hpa.org.uk

Source: Davey P (ed.) (2010) *Medicine at a Glance*, 3rd edn. Reproduced with permission of John Wiley & Sons Ltd.

Figure 20.2 Presenting symptoms and signs in infants and children with UTI

Age group		Symptoms and signs Most common ——————→ Least common		
Infants younger than 3 months		Fever Vomiting Lethargy Irritability	Poor feeding Failure to thrive	Abdominal pain Jaundice Haematuria Offensive urine
Infants and children 3 months or older	Preverbal	Fever	Abdominal pain Loin tenderness Vomiting Poor feeding	Lethargy Irritability Haematuria Offensive urine Failure to thrive
	Verbal	Frequency Dysuria	Dysfunctional voiding Changes to continence Abdominal pain Loin tenderness	Fever Malaise Vomiting Haematuria Offensive urine Cloudy urine

Source: National Institute for Health and Clinical Excellence (2007) CG 54 UTI in children: Urinary tract infection in children: diagnosis, treatment and long-term management. London: NICE. Available from http://guidance.nice.org.uk/CG54. Reproduced with permission

Approach to patient

Urinary tract infections (UTIs) can be distressing but are not usually severe, and a short course of antibiotics is all that is needed. Certain cases, such as men, children, patients with systemic illness and the elderly, may require more in-depth investigations and possible referral.

A good history of symptoms, duration and associated symptoms can give a good indication if a simple urinary infection is likely or a more severe illness.

Always check vital signs and examine the whole of the patient, not just the abdomen.

Specific conditions
Uncomplicated urinary tract infection in women

This is a common presentation. It is more common in females than men owing to the length of the urethra. Common causative pathogens include *Escherichia coli* (90%), *Klebsiella*, *Proteus* and *Enterobacter*.

Usual symptoms include suprapubic pain, urgency, dysuria and frequency.

In the case of a female with two of the above symptoms, a urinary dipstick can be positive for nitrites and leucocytes. In such cases a short course of antibiotics such as trimethoprim 200 mg bd for 3 days can be considered. (See Figure 20.1.)

Urinary microscopy and culture will need to be sent for those with systemic illness, pregnancy, for patients with long-term catheters and recurrent UTIs that do not improve. Discuss difficult cases with microbiology as sensitivity patterns may suggest an alternative antibiotic.

Urinary tract infection in men

Males between the ages of 20 and 60 have a very low incidence of a simple UTI. Differential causes can include prostatitis or epididimytis. Dysuria and frequency may be symptoms of a sexually transmitted disease (see Chapter 21). Some may be caused by a functional or structural problem.

History of urinary symptoms, penile discharge, hesitancy and interrupted flow should be elicited.

Examination may reveal minimal tenderness or a localised tenderness in the abdomen/testicle. Urine dipstick can be carried out; however, a definitive culture is required.

A urine dipstick showing microscopic haematuria should be sent for culture and sensitivity at any age. If no UTI is found then an urgent referral to urology must be made. If a UTI is confirmed then follow-up should be arranged after antibiotic treatment. Repeat urine dipstick should be performed to rule out ongoing haematuria. Recurrent haematuria and frank haematuria require urgent urology outpatient referral.

Treatment should be for 7 days unless the patient is pyrexial, in which case a 2 week antibiotic course should be considered to cover possible prostatic involvement.

Referral to a urologist should be considered, especially for males with recurrent infection or pyrexia from a UTI.

Urinary tract infection in the elderly

Elderly patients with a UTI can present with confusion or new-onset incontinence. Consider culture in those with symptoms. Patients well with asymptomatic positive urine dipstick do not require antibiotics as asymptomatic bacteriuria is common in the elderly.

Paediatric urinary tract infection

Children can present with a variety of symptoms and signs depending upon their age group. Fever, vomiting and poor feeding in the very young are common, while some older children can describe dysuria.

Figure 20.2 illustrates the different symptoms and signs according to age group. Investigations and history vary owing to these age groups.

Treatment of children is guided by the risk of severity of infection as judged by the feverish child guidelines (see Chapter 42). For those with mild symptoms, follow local antibiotic guidelines.

Further investigations are required only if the child is less than 6 months or has an atypical (seriously ill/non-*E. coli* strain/raised creatinine) or recurrent UTI. In such cases referral to a paediatric team for follow-up is appropriate.

Urinary tract infection in pregnancy

A usually uncomplicated UTI in a pregnant woman has an increased likelihood of progressing to pyelonephritis due to the relaxation of the ureteric sphincters.

Treatment with pregnancy-appropriate antibiotics and follow-up of these patients are vital in order to look for and prevent complications. Urine should be sent for culture and sensitivity and local guidance on presumptive antibiotic therapy followed.

Pyelonephritis

Urinary infections can ascend via the ureters, causing infections in the kidney. Patients can present with severe loin pain, pyrexia and other systemic features. Alternative causes can be urinary calculi causing obstruction or a superimposed infection.

Examination can reveal severe loin pain, renal angle tenderness and a positive urine dipstick.

Treatment consists of antibiotics, analgesia and urology referral in many cases, particularly if pre-existing renal disease, immunosuppression (including diabetes) or systemic upset is present. Urine should be sent for culture. Further investigations may be required, such as an ultrasound or computed tomography, if symptoms persist or complications are likely.

 Diagnoses not to be missed

Haematuria

Micro- and macroscopic haematuria may be a sign of malignancy, infection or other renal tract disease. Have a low threshold for arranging follow-up or referral, particularly in painless macroscopic haematuria in older men, as this commonly points to a malignancy.

21 Urogenital problems

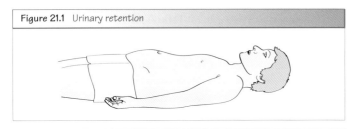

Figure 21.1 Urinary retention

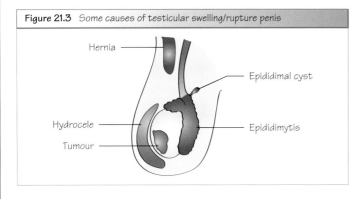

Figure 21.2 Testicular torsion

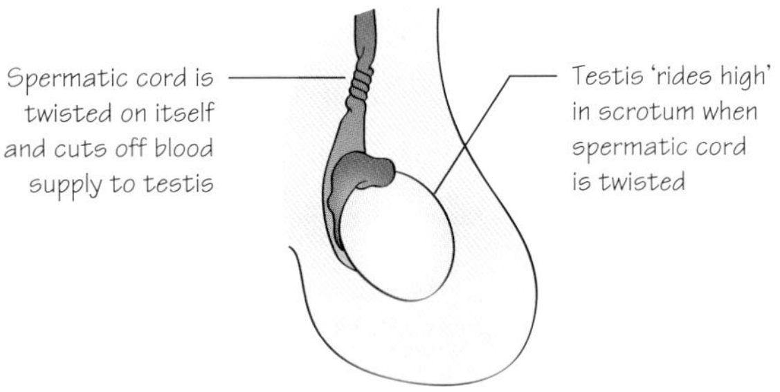

Spermatic cord is twisted on itself and cuts off blood supply to testis

Testis 'rides high' in scrotum when spermatic cord is twisted

Table 21.1 Conditions to consider in the patient with scrotal swelling
Epididymitis
Torsion of epididymal cyst
Hernia
Spermatocele
Hydrocele
Tumour

Figure 21.3 Some causes of testicular swelling/rupture penis

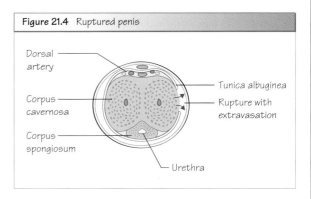

Hernia

Epididimal cyst

Hydrocele

Tumour

Epididimytis

Figure 21.4 Ruptured penis

Dorsal artery

Corpus cavernosa

Corpus spongiosum

Tunica albuginea

Rupture with extravasation

Urethra

Minor Injury and Minor Illness at a Glance, First Edition. Edited by Francis Morris, Jim Wardrope, and Shammi Ramlakhan.

Acute retention of urine

This is a common problem and requires immediate treatment as it is very painful and if the bladder is allowed to distend too much then permanent damage may occur to the bladder wall muscles. The diagnosis is straightforward, with a history of being unable to pass urine, severe pain and a palpable distended bladder (Figure 21.1). Passing a urinary catheter provides immediate relief. Patients should be referred to a urologist for follow-up.

Acute retention in women is much rarer and the causes include neurological problems, drugs side effects and gynaecological problems.

Renal colic

Typical renal colic presents with severe loin pain that radiates to the groin area. Ruptured abdominal aortic aneurism is frequently mis-diagnosed as renal colic and in patients over the age of 55 years it needs to be excluded by non-contrast computed tomography (NCCT).

Note any previous problems with renal colic.
- *Examination.* Check vital signs. Examination of the abdomen is important, especially in older patients. There will usually be evidence of blood (90% sensitive) in the urine on strip testing.
- *Investigation.* This will be decided by local protocol. In younger patients a plain X-ray of the kidneys, ureters and bladder (KUB) may be requested. The absence of a stone on X-ray does not exclude the diagnosis as the test is not very sensitive (44–77%). The imaging method of choice is NCCT, which has a sensitivity of 94–100% for renal calculi. Ultrasound is a cheaper alternative.
- *Treatment.* Analgesia is a priority and the first-line treatment is diclofenac suppository (as long as there are no contra-indications). If the pain settles and there are no signs of ureteric obstruction, many patients can be referred to an outpatient urological clinic for follow-up. If the patient is still in severe pain, is unwell or has systemic signs of infection they will require admission.

Testicular torsion

The diagnosis not to miss is torsion of the testicle. In this condition the vascular pedicle becomes twisted, resulting in necrosis if the problem is not corrected within a few hours (Figure 21.2). It is most common in young men under the age of 30. The pain, usually severe, may be felt in the lower abdomen or hip. The testis is very tender and any movement increases the pain.

Any patient with suspected torsion must be referred immediately to a urologist.

Scrotal swelling/pain

Conditions to be considered are shown in Table 21.1. Ensure that the problem is not a groin hernia that has reached the scrotum. Epididymi-tis is more common in older men. Often there is a history of lower urinary tract symptoms. The epididymis (posterior to the body of the testis) is tender. There may be signs of a urinary tract infection on strip testing. If torsion is excluded, antibiotics are given. The patient should be followed up by their GP.

Painless scrotal swelling may be due to a hydrocele or groin hernia. Tumour is a rare but important cause. All patients with unexplained scrotal swelling should have an ultrasound (see Figure 21.3).

Penile injury and paraphimosis

Paraphimosis is where the retracted foreskin is stuck behind the head of the penis. The diagnosis is obvious. Local cooling with iced water and gentle local pressure usually reduce the swelling of the head of the penis to allow reduction of the foreskin.

Minor tears of the frenulum do not need any treatment.

Rupture of the penis can occur during intercourse. There is immediate loss of erection, pain and marked bruising. Such patients need urgent review by a urologist (Figure 21.4).

Sexually transmitted diseases

These diseases may be asymptomatic but commonly present with urinary tract symptoms, often dysuria or discharge. Other presentations include lower abdominal pain in women and epididymitis in men.

Common organisms include chlamydia, gonococcus and trichomonas. Syphillis and HIV are less common but need to be excluded as patients may have more than one infection.

A history of sexual activity is essential. Swabs should be taken and in men a first-pass urine specimen is also taken. Treatment is with antibiotics. Patients should be referred to a sexual health clinic for follow-up. Contact tracing will be an important part of the work-up.

Patients at high risk of HIV infection may need post-exposure prophylaxis; ask for advice immediately from the local sexual health specialists.

Diagnoses not to be missed

- Suspect rupture of an aortic aneurism in older patients with renal colic type symptoms.
- Any male with sudden-onset severe testicular pain needs immediate referral to a urologist to exclude a torsion of the testis.
- Severe pain and swelling in the penis should be referred to a urologist to exclude rupture of the corpus cavernosum.
- All patients with symptoms of a sexually transmitted disease need referral to a sexual health clinic.
- Discuss patients at high risk of HIV exposure immediately with a sexual health specialist.

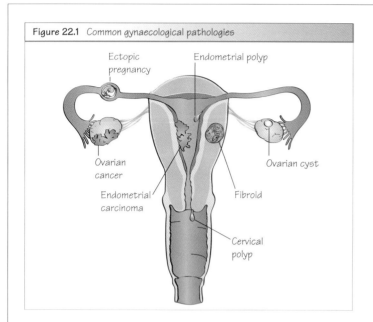

Figure 22.1 Common gynaecological pathologies

Ectopic pregnancy
Endometrial polyp
Ovarian cancer
Endometrial carcinoma
Cervical polyp
Fibroid
Ovarian cyst

Table 22.1 Causes of dysmenorrhea

Adenomyosis – growth of endometrium within the uterine wall
Pelvic inflammatory disease
Endometriosis – endometrial tissue in a site other than the uterine cavity
Irritable bowel syndrome; although not gynaecological, can be exacerbated during menstruation
Congenital abnormalities of the genital tract meaning the menstrual flow is obstructed and builds up in the uterus causing pressure and pain

Table 22.2 Common treatment options in gynaecology

Drug	Mode of action	Indication
Tranexemic acid	Antifibrinolytic, reduces blood loss	Heavy periods
Mefenamic acid	Nonsteroidal anti-inflammatory	Painful periods
Norethisterone	Progestagen	Stop bleeding
Combined oral contraceptive pill	Oestrogen and progestagen	Contraception, heavy periods, painful periods
Progesterone only plll (mini pill)	Progestagen	Contraception
Depot provera	Progesterone injection lasting 12 weeks	Contraception
Mirena coil (intra-uterine system IUS)	Progesterone-impregnated IUCD	Contraception, heavy periods
Morning-after pill	Levonorgestrel or ulipristal	Postcoital contraception

Table 22.3 Causes of intermenstrual/postcoital bleeding

Trauma – any break in the skin, even minor, can bleed
Contraception – irregular bleeding while implant used, Depo-Provera, Mirena and mini pill is normal
Pelvic infections, e.g. chlamydia
Cervical pathology – ectropion, carcinoma
Polyps – cervical or endometrial
Fibroids

 Red flags

- Assume all women of child-bearing age are pregnant
- Consider ectopic pregnancy with abdominal pain/early pregnancy bleeding
- Do not forget cervicalc ancer in intramenstrual/postcoital bleeding

Approach to patient
Key skills
• *Menstrual history.* Date of last period, time between periods, how long each period lasts and if heavy or painful.
• *Obstetric history.* How many previous pregnancies? The outcome of each pregnancy (miscarriage, normal vaginal birth, ectopic pregnancy, caesarean section)? Gravidity is the total number of times the patient has been pregnant. Parity is often recorded as P2+2, meaning the woman has had two pregnancies beyond 24 weeks and two miscarriages.
• *Sexual history.* Current relationship, use of contraception or intrauterine contraceptive device (IUCD), any previous sexually transmitted disease, any pain during intercourse (dyspareunia).
• *Gynaecological examination.* Involves an abdominal examination, vaginal and speculum examinations. The timing of the vaginal examinations will depend on a number of factors, including the urgency, the availability of proper facilities, light and equipment. A chaperone is always required. If it is likely that the patient is going to be referred to a gynaecologist urgently, then it might be best to defer.
• *Investigations. Urinalysis* is a simple and quick test that helps diagnose a urinary tract infection, looking for the presence of nitrites, leucocytes and blood. *A urine* **pregnancy test is essential in any woman of child-bearing age with gynaecological symptoms or abdominal pain**. The test is positive within a few days of implantation of the embryo, but a negative urine test does not completely rule out a very early pregnancy.
Vaginal and cervical swabs are needed investigate vaginal discharge or some cases of abdominal pain.
Ultrasound scans (USSs) can be performed either transabdominally or transvaginally (probe inserted into the vagina), therefore obtaining a better view of the uterus and adenexa.

Abdominal pain with a positive pregnancy test
Presume all women of child bearing age are pregnant until proven otherwise.

Ectopic pregnancy can present in many ways from 'classical' sudden collapse with shock, abdominal pain and vaginal bleeding, shoulder tip pain, signs of peritonism to a well patient with minor abdominal pain with no vaginal bleeding. Patients still die from misdiagnosis of this condition. **Abdominal pain in early pregnancy is due to an ectopic pregnancy until proven otherwise**.

Discuss with the gynaecology team. If the patient is well then they may make arrangements to see the patient in the next available early pregnancy assessment unit (EPAU). If the patient is unwell or the bleeding is severe, they will see the patient immediately.

Abdominal pain with a negative pregnancy test
Women can suffer from any of the conditions causing abdominal pain in men, including appendicitis, renal colic, urinary tract infection, biliary and bowel problems. Specific causes include period pain, ovarian cyst rupture or torsion, pelvic inflammatory disease and endometriosis.

Vaginal bleeding in pregnancy
Think of ectopic pregnancy or miscarriage (see earlier).

Miscarriage or spontaneous abortion is the loss of a pregnancy before 24 weeks' gestation. This is common, especially before 12 weeks' gestation. In most cases no specific treatment is required, but the patient should be seen in the EPAU. Rarely, the bleeding can be very heavy. If there are signs of major blood loss then urgent gynaecological admission may be required.

Significant vaginal bleeding in later pregnancy needs referral as an emergency to the labour ward.

Period problems
Amenorrhoea
Lack of periods can be primary (never had periods) or secondary (had periods but stopped).
• *Assessment.* Take a full medical and gynaecological history and examine the patient. Do a pregnancy test. Check thyroid function. This is rarely an urgent problem. Refer to GP.

Oligomenorrhoea
Infrequent periods; the investigation and treatment are similar to amenorrhoea.

Menorrhagia
Abnormally heavy and/or prolonged periods. Usually 'dysfunctional'; other causes include clotting disorders, idiopathic thrombocytopenic purpura, Von Willebrand's disease or anticoagulant medication, and uterine pathology such as fibroids or carcinoma.
• *Investigation.* Do a pregnancy test. A full blood count and clotting screen may be needed. Refer to GP for further investigation.
• *Treatment.* Initially try tranexamic acid and mefenamic acid. Other options include the combined oral contraceptive pill (COCP) or a Mirena coil or endometrial ablation.

Dysmenorrhoea
Painful periods; often no investigation is needed, just pain relief.
• *Examination.* USS, swabs – antibiotics if positive, laparoscopy if endometriosis suspected, COCP.

Intermenstrual bleeding
Bleeding in between periods and **postcoital bleeding** – bleeding after sexual intercourse. If mid cycle, intermenstrual bleeding can be normal and associated with ovulation.
• *Investigation.* Examination, swabs, USS, smear test.
• *Treatment.* Change of or commencing contraception – COCP.

► **Diagnoses not to be missed**

• Assume all women of child-bearing age are pregnant.
• Ectopic pregnancy can be a difficult diagnosis; always consider in a woman presenting with abdominal pain/and or early pregnancy bleeding.
• Do not forget cervical cancer as a cause of intramenstrual/postcoital bleeding, especially if a woman has not had regular cervical smears.

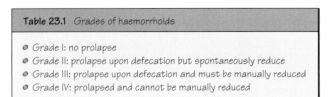

Table 23.1 Grades of haemorrhoids

- Grade I: no prolapse
- Grade II: prolapse upon defecation but spontaneously reduce
- Grade III: prolapse upon defecation and must be manually reduced
- Grade IV: prolapsed and cannot be manually reduced

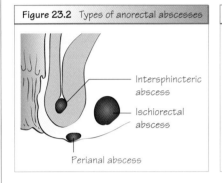

Figure 23.2 Types of anorectal abscesses

Intersphincteric abscess

Ischiorectal abscess

Perianal abscess

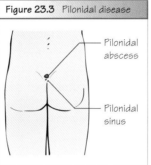

Figure 23.3 Pilonidal disease

Pilonidal abscess

Pilonidal sinus

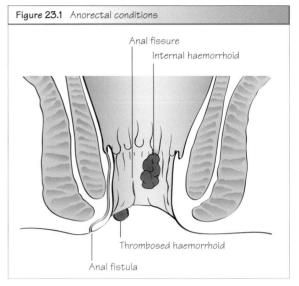

Figure 23.1 Anorectal conditions

Anal fissure

Internal haemorrhoid

Thrombosed haemorrhoid

Anal fistula

Minor Injury and Minor Illness at a Glance, First Edition. Edited by Francis Morris, Jim Wardrope, and Shammi Ramlakhan.

Approach to the patient

Patients with anorectal disorders often present with rectal bleeding, pain or less commonly swelling, itching or discharge. The spectrum of disease is wide and includes perianal manifestations of systemic diseases, sexually transmitted infections, inflammatory bowel disease and malignancy.

The history should elicit the onset and duration of symptoms, relation to defaecation, altered bowel habit and sexual history. Other manifestations suggesting systemic disease, such as pyrexia, recurrence, symptoms of anaemia or weight loss, should also be elicited. Recurrence can indicate an underlying condition such as diabetes, malignancy or immunosuppression.

Examination is undertaken usually with the patient in the lateral position. Inspection for swelling, discharge, induration, erythema or lesions suggestive of a sexually transmitted infection is important. Palpation for tenderness and a rectal examination are also useful, although the latter may be too painful in conditions such as anal fissures, abscesses or thrombosed haemorrhoids. The rectal examination may be normal in cases of haemorrhoids.

Specific conditions
Haemorrhoids

These are thought to be enlarged vascular cushions in the anal canal which are related to straining at stool. Patients usually present with painless passage of bright red blood into the toilet or on wiping. Pain usually means that a complication such as a thrombosed haemorrhoid is present. The grades of haemorrhoids are shown in Figure 23.1. External haemorrhoids can cause itching and discharge.

Most patients can be managed with a high-fibre diet, and although many topical formulations are available, there is little evidence that they are beneficial.

Patients who have profuse bleeding should be appropriately resuscitated and referred to a surgical team.

Thrombosed haemorrhoids

These present with anal pain and purplish swelling. Most can be managed conservatively with ice, stool softeners and analgesia, especially if they present after 48 h. Symptoms usually resolve within 2 weeks. Referral for excision is necessary for necrotic or fourth-degree haemorrhoids.

Patients should be followed up in primary care or surgical outpatient clinics for higher degrees of haemorrhoids.

Anal fissure

This is a superficial tear in the mucosa of the anal verge. It causes significant pain on passage of stool which may last up to 1–2 h afterwards. Small amounts of bright red blood may be seen on wiping. The majority of fissures are in the posterior midline, and an anal skin tag may also be present at the area.

Most anal fissures will heal spontaneously with a high-fibre diet and stool softeners. Symptomatic relief with sitz baths may be useful. Chronic fissures can be treated with topical glyceryl trinitrate or calcium channel blockers. Patients should be followed up in primary care, with failed treatment warranting outpatient surgical referral.

Anal abscesses

These usually form as a result of cryptoglandular infection. Patients present with pain or swelling which is worse on sitting or passing stool. Depending on the location of the abscess, patients may complain of deep anal pain. Perianal abscesses can usually be seen as swelling or erythema with tenderness around the anal verge and buttocks, although deeper abscesses may not have externally visible signs. Patients may be systemically unwell.

Patients with symptoms suggestive of an anal abscess but without externally visible/palpable signs may require imaging to look for deeper seated abscesses, and a low threshold for referral should be maintained.

All patients with anal abscesses should be acutely referred for surgical drainage.

Anal fistulae

Chronic or recurrent abscesses can lead to fistula formation as the abscess tracks and discharges. They cause mostly inflammatory symptoms, such as prurits ani, discharge and skin irritation, although, if blocked, painful abscesses can form.

Surgical treatment is necessary and referral for planned incision is usually acceptable.

Pilonidal disease

This condition is more common in young men, with natal hair playing a role in its development. It occurs in the natal (sacrococcygeal) cleft, and presents with a painful swelling/abscess or in some cases a discharging sinus.

Incision is usually required, and this can be performed under local anaesthetic. Care must be taken to remove all hair fragments from the area. Follow-up is required until resolution, although recurrence is common.

> ## ▶ Diagnoses not to be missed
>
> ### Rectal bleeding
>
> Rectal bleeding in patients over 40 years old should always be investigated for lower gastrointestinal malignancy as a cause. Referral to a surgical clinic for endoscopy is mandatory.
>
> ### Systemic disease
>
> Several systemic diseases may present with perianal symptoms; for example, 20% of patients with Crohn's disease have perianal disease, including multiple fistulae, abscesses and inflammation. Patients with diabetes or immunosuppression may present with recurrent abscesses. In all of these a high index of suspicion for further investigation should be maintained.

Figure 24.1 The Canadian C-spine rule

The Canadian C-spine Rule
For alert (GCS score=15) and stable trauma
patients when cervical spine injury is a concern

1. Any high-risk factor that
   mandates radiography?
   Age ≥ 65 y or
   Dangerous mechanism* or
   Paresthesies in extrememities

   ↓ No

2. Any low-risk factor that allows safe
   assessment of range of motion
   Simple rear-end MVC# or
   Sitting position in ED or
   Ambulatory at any time or
   Delayed onset of neck pain‡ or
   Absence of midline cervical spine
   tenderness

   ↓ Yes

3. Able to actively rotate neck?
   45 degrees left and right

   ↓ Able

   No radiography

→ Radiography

* Dangerous mechanism
• Fall from elevation ≥ 3 ft/5 stairs
• Axial load to head, e.g. diving
• MVC high speed (>100 km/h),
  rollover, ejection
• Motorised recreational vehicles
• Bicycle crash

Simple rear-end MVC excludes
• Pushed into oncoming traffic
• Hit by bus/large truck
• Rollover
• Hit by high-speed vehicle

‡ Delayed
• i.e. not immediate onset of
  neck pain

Source: Bandiera G et al. Ann Emerg Med 2003; 24(3): 395–402
Reproduced with permission from Elsevier

Figure 24.3 Body map of dermatomes

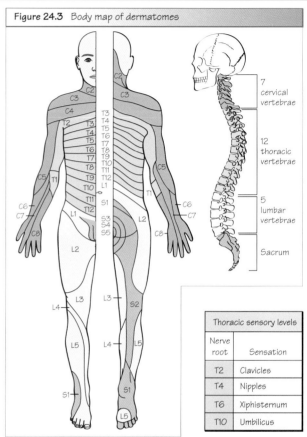

7 cervical vertebrae

12 thoracic vertebrae

5 lumbar vertebrae

Sacrum

Thoracic sensory levels	
Nerve root	Sensation
T2	Clavicles
T4	Nipples
T6	Xiphisternum
T10	Umbilicus

Figure 24.2 Measuring lumbar spine flexion, normal > 7 cm

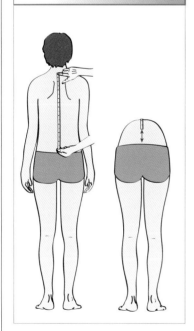

Table 24.1 Dermatomes and myotomes of the upper limb

Nerve root	Reflex	Muscles	Sensation
C5	Biceps	Deltoid/biceps	Lateral upper arm
C6	Brachioradialis/biceps	Wrist extensors/biceps	Lateral foream
C7	Triceps	Wrist flexors, finger extensors, Triceps	Middle finger
C8	–	Finger flexion	Sensation to little finger
T1/2	–	Intrinsic muscles of the hand	Medial arm

Figure 24.4

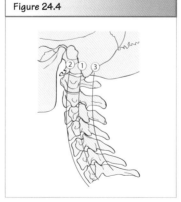

Table 24.2 Dermatomes and myotomes of the lower limb

Nerve root	Reflex	Motor	Sensation
T12, L1,2,3	–	Hip flexion	L1 groin, L2 medial thigh, L3 medial knee
L2,3,4	–	Knee extension	L2 medial thigh, L3 medial knee, L4 Medial mallous
L4	Patella jerk	Ankle dorsiflexion	Medial malleolus
L5	Ankle jerk	Toe extension	Dorsum of foot
S1	Ankle jerk	Ankle plantar flexion	Lateral malleolus and plantar surface of foot
S2,3,4	Anal reflex	Anal wink	Dermatomes around anus

Approach to patient

Use a structured look, feel, move approach, *except* in a patient with a history of significant injury, where the movement section is deliberately omitted until possible unstable injuries have been excluded.

Observe how the patient walks. Do they appear in distress from the pain? How are the holding themselves?

Check temperature and pulse rate.

Some patients brought by ambulance may be immobilised using a collar/bags/tape/spinal board. There are guidelines on how to 'clinically clear the spine'; see Figure 24.1.

Look

In the neck you should note if the normal lordosis (forward curve) is present. Is the neck held normally or pulled to one side as in torticollis? In the thoracic and lumbar spine you should look for scoliosis (curve to one side) and the normal kyphosis (backwards curve) in thoracic area and lordosis in the lumbar area.

Signs of trauma may be noted, such as cuts, grazes and bruises. Lipoma-like swelling or patches of hair on the lower back may be a sign of spina bifida.

Feel

The entire spine should be palpated noting where painful. C7/T1 are the most prominent spinous processes, and the L4/5 junction is at about the level of the iliac crests. Spinous processes should all be inline. Approximately 2.5 cm lateral to the spinous process is the facet joint. Finally, paraspinal muscles should be palpated, noting any tenderness or muscle spasm.

Movement
Cervical spine

If there are any concerns of cervical spine trauma, neck range of motion should not be performed until the neck has been cleared. Otherwise neck active movements should be observed. The neck typically has around 80° of rotation in each direction; lateral flexion is about 45°. Flexion and extension are about 75° and 60° each.

Thoracic spine

The thoracic spine is relatively immobile; its primary movement is rotation.

Lumbar spine

Measure flexion as indicated in Figure 24.2. Check lateral flexion and extension.

Neurological examination

A through neurological examination is part of any spinal examination. It should include assessment of power, tone, reflexes and sensation in both the upper and lower limbs. See Figure 24.3, Tables 24.1 and 24.2 for the sensory and motor distribution of the nerve roots.

Special tests
Sciatic nerve stretch test

Keeping the knee extended, flex the hip (lift up the straight leg). If pain occurs and shoots from the back down the leg below the knee it is suggestive of compression of the sciatic nerve (L4, L5, S1). Slightly lowering the leg and the dorsi-flexing the foot will again bring on the pain. You need to be carful not to confuse this pain with that of a tight hamstring.

Rectal examination

Assessment of the peripheral nervous system requires Per rectum examination to be complete. Perianal sensation should be documented as well as tone. In the superficial anal reflex, touching the perianal skin should cause the anus to contract.

Abdominal examination and pulses

The examinations are mandatory in the elderly but good practice in all patients with back pain. Aortic aneurism will be missed if you do not look for it.

X-rays

In non-traumatic back and neck pain, X-rays are not indicated unless there are "red flag" symptoms or neurological signs. If there is a history of significant trauma, x-rays are indicated.

Use the ABCS system to interpret the images:
- A – adequacy and alignment. Can you see to the upper part of the body of the T1 vertebra? Check the alignment of the anterior and posterior aspects of the vertebral bodies and the spinous processes and the spinal processes (Figure 24.4).
- B – bones. Check all the bones, especially the odontoid peg.
- C – cartilaginous spaces. Check the disc spaces and the gaps between the spinous processes.
- S – soft tissues. Check the width of the soft tissue shadows anterior to the vertebral bodies (cervical spine) and the paravertebral stripe.

> ### ▶ Diagnoses not to be missed
>
> Consider infection (e.g. discitis, osteomyelitis) or bony metastases in any patient with new onset or worsening constant non-traumatic neck or back pain, particularly if night pain is a feature. Such a history, especially if associated with localised tenderness and/or swelling of the spine on examination, is an indication for further investigation; for example, imaging and inflammatory markers.

Figure 25.1 Performing a log roll

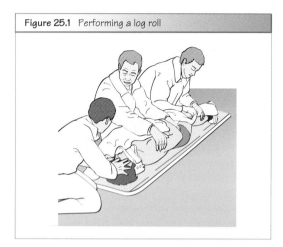

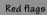

Red flags

- History of major trauma (or minor trauma in the elderly)
- Extremes of age (< 20 or > 55)
- Systemic symptoms (weight loss, fevers, chills)
- History of malignancy
- Night pain
- Intravenous drug use
- Immunocompromised (HIV, chemotherapy, etc.)
- Chronic steroid use
- Rheumatoid arthritis/ankylosing spondylitis
- Significant/progressive neurological signs
- Bladder or bowel dysfunction

Figure 25.2 Whiplash occurs during rear-end vehicle collision

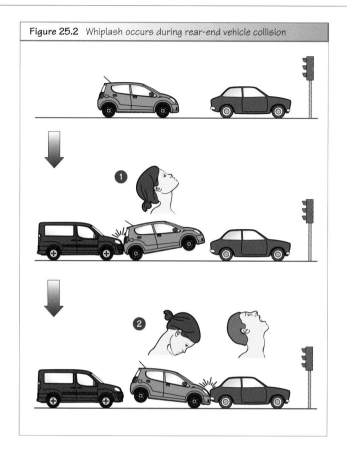

Diagnosis – trauma and non-trauma

Neck injuries are a common cause of attendance to the emergency department. The majority of these are simple sprains caused by motor vehicle collisions, but the effects of missing a significant problem and causing quadriplegia are catastrophic.

• *History.* Has the patient had an injury or is the problem non-traumatic? If traumatic, then establish the exact mechanism. Falls >1 m, diving accidents and severe RTCs are the commonest causes of fracture. Ask about neurological symptoms. A history of rheumatoid arthritis or ankylosing spondylitis should raise the index of suspicion. In non-trauma a full history is important.

• *Examination.* All patients need a thorough neurological examination to include power, tone, sensation and reflexes. Patients should have their whole spine examined, in the case of trauma this needs to be done in a controlled way to protect the potentially injured spine (see Figure 25.1).

• *Investigations.* Will depend on the history. The C-spine decision rules can significantly reduce the need for X-ray in minor rear-end shunts (see Figure 24.1). For other mechanisms, plain X-rays will probably be required. Those with abnormal neurological signs or significant ongoing symptoms following normal plain radiographs need further imaging (computed tomography (CT) or magnetic resonance imaging), and orthopaedic referral is often warranted.

• *Interpretation.* C-spine X-ray interpretation is assisted by using the ABCS system: A – check adequacy (can you see C7/T1 junction) and alignment; B – examine the bones; C – cartilaginous spaces between the vertebrae and the spinous processes; S – look at the soft tissues (see Chapter 24).

Acute neck sprain

Commonly known as 'whiplash' injuries and are often caused by rear-end motor vehicle collision (Figure 25.2).

Pain and stiffness are often delayed and may take up to 48 h to be at their maximum. There is often associated back/shoulder pain (particularly inter-scapular), headache, and pins and needles in the arms.

Examination reveals often diffuse tenderness all over the neck, especially in the paravertebral muscles. If there is isolated bony tenderness, significant pain on movement or inability to rotate to 45°, X-rays are required.

Advise early mobilisation and simple analgesics (paracetamol/nonsteroidal anti-inflammatory drugs (NSAIDs)) with weak opiates if required. Avoid the use of soft collars. Give an advice leaflet and outline red flag symptoms and when to seek further medical advice.

Other trauma

Patients with more significant mechanisms, especially falls over a metre (e.g. down stairs), diving and rugby accidents, motorcycle/bicycle/pedestrian road traffic accidents, will need proper imaging; this may need CT.

Cervical spine fractures

These are relatively uncommon and generally require a significant mechanism to occur. They should all be treated as being unstable and so be immobilised and referred to orthopaedics/spinal surgery for further assessment.

Non-trauma torticollis

Also known as wry neck, this is caused by a 'slipped cervical disc' or facet joint dysfunction that leads to painful spasm of the sternocleido-mastoid or trapezius muscle. The patient is usually young and presents with the head over to the affected side.

It can occur on sudden movement of the neck to one side or the patient may awake with it. It can be secondary to another pathology local infection/inflammation in the neck and cervical spine injury.

Treatment of torticollis is with simple analgesics including NSAIDs. If spasm is severe then a short course of a benzodiazepine (e.g. diazepam) may be required to aid muscle relaxation. Some patients find that local heat (e.g. hot water bottle) helps with symptoms. Most cases of torticollis resolve within 5–10 days.

Osteoarthritis and disc prolapse

Neck pain and stiffness due to degenerative disease of the cervical spine is very common, and incidence increases with age. Acute disc prolapse can cause similar problems as in the lumbar spine, such as severe pain, pressure on nerve roots causing neurological symptoms in the limbs or pressure on the spinal cord potentially causing paraplegia.

A careful history and detailed neurological examination are required.

Where there are no signs or symptoms of abnormal neurology in the upper or lower limbs, then advise simple exercises, adequate analgesia and advice on when to seek further medical review.

Rarer diagnoses and non-spinal causes of neck pain

Spinal infections and tumours are rare causes of neck pain (see Chapter 'red flags' for these conditions).

Severe throat infections and retropharyngeal abscess may cause severe neck pain and spasm.

Patients with rheumatoid arthritis and ankylosing spondylitis can fracture their spines with minimal trauma.

Table 26.1 Causes of back pain

Musculo-skeletal	Fractures	Infection	Radiation abdomen	Radiation chest
Facet joints	Trauma	Spine	Aortic aneurism	Pulmonary emboli
Ligaments	Osteoporotic	Kidney	Pancreatitis	Pneumonia
Intervertebral disc	Pathological		Pathological	Myocardial infarction

Table 26.2 Red flag symptoms in back pain history

- History of major trauma (or minor trauma in the elderly)
- Extremes of age (< 20 or > 55)
- Systemic symptoms (weight loss, fevers, chills)
- History of malignancy
- Night pain
- Intravenous drug use
- Immunocompromised (HIV, chemotherapy, etc.)
- Chronic steroid use
- Significant/progressive neurological signs
- Bladder or bowel dysfunction

Table 26.3 When patients need to seek immediate advice

Bladder disturbance
Bowel incontinence
Perineal numbness
New sexual dysfunction
Progressive leg weakness
Bilateral leg symptoms

Figure 26.1 Intervertebral discs bulge posteriorly into the spinal canal

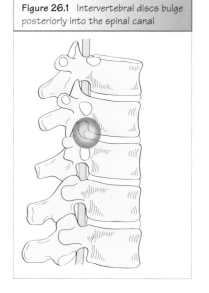

Minor Injury and Minor Illness at a Glance, First Edition. Edited by Francis Morris, Jim Wardrope, and Shammi Ramlakhan.

64 © 2014 John Wiley & Sons, Ltd. Published 2014 by John Wiley & Sons, Ltd. Companion Website: www.ataglanceseries.com/minorinjury

Back pain affects about 30% of population each year. The majority of back pain seen in minor illness settings does not have a serious pathology; however, you need to be careful not to miss a serious condition.

Table 26.1 lists many of the possible causes of back pain. 'Mechanical back pain' is by far the commonest cause. Such pain originates from the small joints of the spine or from the intervertebral discs. The pain can be severe and debilitating. See 'Diagnoses not to be missed'.

Approach to the patient

• *History.* This is the best tool you have to alert you to the possibility of a 'serious diagnosis not to be missed'. Table 26.2 lists the features in the history (red flags) that merit investigation and referral for further care. This section does not deal with traumatic back pain.
• *Age.* This is an important discriminator. Simple back pain is uncommon in children, and in older patients serious conditions are more common.
• *Cancer and sepsis.* These conditions when involving the spine can be difficult diagnoses. Night pain, systemic symptoms, immunodeficiency, previous cancer or intravenous drug abuse are clues that need further investigation.
• *Neurological symptoms.* Symptoms such as leg weakness or problems with bladder and bowel function can indicate pressure on the nerve roots.
• *Examination.* See Chapter 24. Remember, look, feel, move, neurological exam (including per rectal (PR)), abdomen and pulses.
• *Investigation.* In a typical case of mechanical back pain with no red flag symptoms plain X-rays are not required (unless the pain has been going on for more than 6 weeks). Magnetic resonance imaging (MRI) is becoming the imaging of choice if serious pathology is suspected.

Mechanical back pain

• *Diagnosis.* This diagnosis is made after other more serious causes of back pain have been excluded; patients tend to be young (20–40 years) complaining of lower back pain. A sudden movement such as twisting or overreaching often initiates these acute episodes. Pain is exacerbated by movement and improves with rest. The patient often has difficulty moving. Spinal movements are very much reduced. You may find some para-spinal tenderness and more rarely muscle spasm. There should be no neurological signs.
• *Plan.* The patient should be encouraged to manage their own condition. There is clear evidence that 'keeping moving' is much better than rest. Initially, advise simple analgesics (paracetamol/nonsteroidal anti-inflammatory drugs), more severe cases will need a weak opioid (e.g. codeine). In severe spasm a short course of diazepam may be beneficial. Some patients feel that local heat or cold help with their pain.
• *Communication and follow-up.* The patient should be provided with an advice leaflet showing exercises to improve their back pain, along with a list of red flag symptoms of when to seek further medical advice (see Table 24.3). Of those who require time off work, most will be back within 1 week. Patients who require longer should be referred by their GP for an exercise programme.

Sciatica/prolapsed disc

True sciatica is caused by pressure on the nerve roots that make up the sciatic nerve (L4–S2). The pain typically goes below the knee. Straight-leg raising and sciatic nerve stretch tests are positive (see Chapter 24). If there is no objective neurological deficit or the deficit is confined to a single nerve root, then provide the usual advice for back pain and arrange careful follow-up with GP within one week. Most cases resolve within 6 weeks. If there are multiple nerve roots involved, bilateral symptoms and signs of bladder or bowel problems, refer urgently for further investigation.

Cauda equina syndrome

This is a neurological emergency where pressure on the nerve roots in the lower part of the spinal canal causes neurological dysfunction. Causes include large central disc prolapse, metastatic/primary tumours, or bony fragments/haematoma in trauma (see Figure 26.1).

This condition usually presents acutely, but onset may be gradual. Symptoms include bilateral leg/back pain and weakness in both legs, altered perianal sensation (saddle anaesthesia), sphincter disturbance (urinary/faecal incontinence and retention) and sudden sexual dysfunction. You are likely to find lower motor neurone weakness. PR examination will reveal reduced/absent perianal sensation and reduced anal tone.

All patients with concerns of possible cauda equina should be referred as an inpatient for further investigation (usually MRI). Urgent surgery is required if the patient is to recover function; however, sphincter problems often persist and recovery is not full.

Diagnoses not to be missed

Back pain in the elderly

Significant and serious pathology is more common. Wedge fractures of the vertebral body may occur with minimal or no trauma. Cancer and infection are more common. Have a low threshold for obtaining X-rays.

Abdominal causes of back pain

A number of intra-abdominal pathologies can cause back pain. Renal colic classically causes unilateral back pain that radiates to the groin; this pain comes and goes in waves and can be associated with nausea and vomiting. The pain in pancreatitis is classically central abdominal and radiates to the back; patients generally are nauseous and vomit.

The most serious cause of intra-abdominal back pain is a leaking aortic aneurysm. This again causes pain that radiates through to the back; the patient may be shocked if significant blood loss has occurred. Many senior emergency department clinicians are able to ultrasound to look for an aortic aneurysm; this, however, will not tell you if it is leaking. Urgent resuscitation and referral to a vascular surgeon are essential.

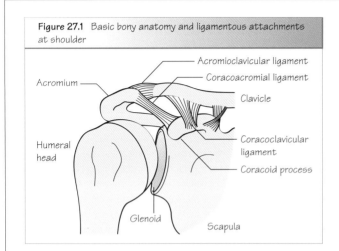

Figure 27.1 Basic bony anatomy and ligamentous attachments at shoulder

Acromioclavicular ligament
Coracoacromial ligament
Acromium
Clavicle
Humeral head
Coracoclavicular ligament
Coracoid process
Glenoid
Scapula

Figure 27.2 The 'painful arc'

180°
170°
120°
Painless
Glenohumeral painful arc
45–60°
Painless

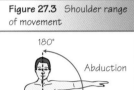

Figure 27.3 Shoulder range of movement

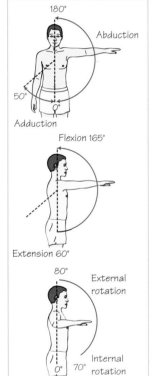

180°
Abduction
50°
Adduction

Flexion 165°
Extension 60°

80°
External rotation
0°
70°
Internal rotation

Figure 27.4 Resisted abduction

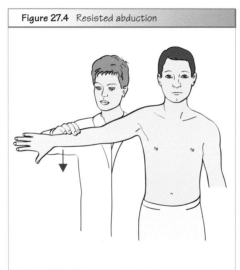

Figure 27.5 Resisted internal rotation

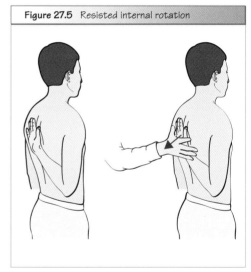

The shoulder girdle is where the upper limbs join the axial skeleton. There are a number of joints, notably the glenohumeral, the scapulo-thoracic, acromioclavicular and sternoclavicular joints, supported by strong ligamentous attachments and muscle groups that interact to allow a complex range of movements (Figure 27.1). Problems with the shoulder may have a profound impact upon activities of daily living, such as hair washing, getting dressed and sleeping, as well as restricting sporting activities.

Approach to the patient

When examining a patient with a suspected shoulder injury it is important to consider possible associated injury to the head, neck or chest that would need more urgent attention. Ensure that the patient has been offered analgesia before proceeding with clinical examination. Exposure of both shoulders and upper torso is required for an adequate examination, and so an appropriately private setting must be selected. In some circumstances a chaperone may be required.

In the absence of a history of injury, soft tissue problems should be considered, but some medical problems can result in pain referred to the shoulder. Ischaemic chest pain, diaphragmatic irritation from pneumonia and blood within the peritoneum from, for example, an ectopic pregnancy can produce shoulder tip pain.

Examination

Examination follows a 'look, feel, move, special tests' approach and should include consideration of the joint above (neck) and below (elbow) and a neurovascular examination.

Look

Look for bony deformities, such as a prominent sternoclavicular joint (subluxation), swelling over the clavicle (new or old fracture) and prominent acromioclavicular joint (partial or complete ligamentous disruption); a 'squared off' appearance of the shoulder suggests anterior glenohumeral dislocation, and muscle wasting may be present.

Ask the patient to indicate areas of specific tenderness.

Feel

Palpate systematically, comparing the affected side with the non-affected side and assess for tenderness and palpable deformity.

Start at the centre at the sternoclavicular joint and then move laterally across the clavicle palpating the acromioclavicular joint.

Palpate the glenohumeral joint anteriorly and laterally and the head of the biceps anteriorly.

Pain from injuries to the clavicle and the acromioclavicular joint are well localised, though pain from rotator cuff injuries and glenohumeral joint injuries is often experienced over the lateral side of the upper arm. Pain from the neck is usually experienced across the top of the shoulder and may radiate down the lateral border of the upper arm.

Move

Remember to assess symmetry of movement with the unaffected side. Assess active (patient-initiated) movements and, when painful or limited, passive (examiner-initiated) movements. Full active and passive ranges of movement increase the likelihood that the injury is confined to the soft tissue.

Normal range of movement

• **Abduction: 0–170°.** Abduction past 90° involves the rotation of the scapula (scapulo-thoracic) and is not a movement confined to the glenohumeral joint. Difficulties in initiating abduction suggest supraspinatus pathology, but passive movements are generally unaffected. The deltoid is the prime mover for abduction after the initial 20°, so that the patient can actively abduct in the presence of a supraspinatus tear if abduction is *initiated* passively. A painful range of movement between approximately 60 and 120° (the 'painful arc'; Figure 27.2) is associated with impingement of the supraspinatus on the acromion. A decrease in both active and passive movements is seen in adhesive capsulitis ('frozen shoulder').
• **Adduction: 0–50°.** Test by touching the front of the opposite shoulder with the hand.
• **Flexion (forward movement of the arm): 0–165°.**
• **Extension (backward movement of the arm): 0–60°.**
• **Internal and external rotations: 0–70° and 0–80° respectively.** Internal and external rotations are often assessed with the upper arm held abducted at 90° (Figure 27.3). If this is not possible because of restricted abduction the arms can be held in front of the body with the elbows flexed at 90°. In this position internal rotation is achieved by moving the hand across the body, and external rotation by moving it away from the body. A further test for internal rotation involves the patient placing the dorsum of their hand on their back in the midline and reaching as high up their back as they can with their upturned hand; touching between T8 and T5 is considered normal.

Special tests

Dynamic tests of the individual muscle components of the rotator cuff can identify individual tendon injuries.
• **Supraspinatus.** With the arm held straight, the shoulder in forward flexion of 30° and thumbs pointing down to the ground, the patient is asked to abduct the arm against resistance, which is painful when pathology is present (Figure 27.4).
• **Infraspinatus and teres minor.** There is pain and/or restriction of resisted external rotation of the glenohumeral joint.
• **Subscapularis.** The dorsum of the hand is placed against the back in the mid-lumbar region (internal rotation). The patient will experience pain or restriction of movement on attempts to internally rotate further by lifting their hand off their back against resistance (Figure 27.5).

Completing the examination

Distal neurovascular examination should include testing of the radial, median and ulnar nerves, the axillary nerve and assessment of the radial pulses.

Investigation

Shoulder X-rays consist of two views: the anterior–posterior and lateral or axial view. Many clinicians find the axial views easier to interpret, particularly with reference to whether the shoulder is in joint or not.

When the injury is confined to the *acromioclavicular* joint, specific X-rays of this joint should be requested.

28 Shoulder injuries

Box 28.1 Clinical features of an anterior shoulder dislocation

- 'Squared off' appearance of shoulder
- Palpable gap below acromion
- The humeral head is palpable inferior to the glenoid
- All movements of the glenohumoral joint are very limited/absent

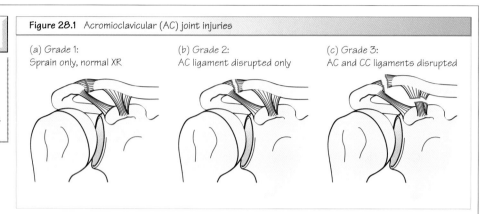

Figure 28.1 Acromioclavicular (AC) joint injuries

(a) Grade 1:
Sprain only, normal XR

(b) Grade 2:
AC ligament disrupted only

(c) Grade 3:
AC and CC ligaments disrupted

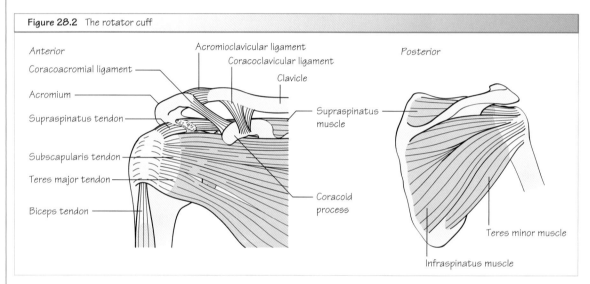

Figure 28.2 The rotator cuff

Anterior

Coracoacromial ligament
Acromium
Supraspinatus tendon
Subscapularis tendon
Teres major tendon
Biceps tendon

Acromioclavicular ligament
Coracoclavicular ligament
Clavicle
Coracoid process

Posterior

Supraspinatus muscle
Teres minor muscle
Infraspinatus muscle

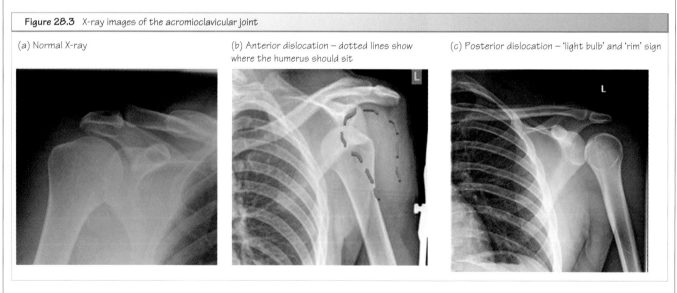

Figure 28.3 X-ray images of the acromioclavicular joint

(a) Normal X-ray

(b) Anterior dislocation – dotted lines show where the humerus should sit

(c) Posterior dislocation – 'light bulb' and 'rim' sign

Minor Injury and Minor Illness at a Glance, First Edition. Edited by Francis Morris, Jim Wardrope, and Shammi Ramlakhan.

The glenohumeral joint is highly mobile owing to the 3:1 ratio in size between the humeral head and the glenoid cavity. This affords great mobility but an increased susceptibility to injury. Strong ligamentous attachments and the rotator cuff muscles stabilise the joint and maintain the correct position of the humeral head during movement. Nevertheless, 10% of sporting injuries and more than half of large joint dislocations involve the shoulder.

Specific injuries

Acromioclavicular joint injury

This occurs typically in young, active males, after a direct blow or fall onto the outermost part of the shoulder with the arm adducted.

Examination reveals point tenderness over the acromioclavicular joint. An X-ray may show separation of the joint. Injuries are graded (Figure 28.1). Grade 1: minimal or no separation on X-ray. There is a sprain or partial tear of the acromioclavicular ligament. Grade 2: there is complete rupture of the acromioclavicular ligament and subluxation of the joint. Grade 3: the coracoclavicular ligaments are also torn, and there is complete separation of the distal end of the clavicle from the acromion.

Grade 1 injuries are treated by analgesia and/or broad arm sling. Grade 2 and 3 injuries should be referred to the fracture clinic.

Clavicle fracture

This results from a direct blow or fall onto an outstretched hand, resulting in localised pain, swelling and/or deformity; 80% involve the middle third of the clavicle and 15% the distal third. Displacement is limited by the integrity of the coracoclavicular ligament.

Management is usually conservative, with a broad arm sling with follow-up in the fracture clinic. Surgery is *considered* in fractures with separation *and* comminution, if skin is threatened or if there is neurovascular involvement.

Anterior glenohumeral dislocation

Dislocation is usually the result of a fall onto an arm which is forced into abduction, external rotation and extension, giving rise to marked pain and deformity. See Box 28.1.

X-ray and a full neurovascular examination including axillary nerve assessment should be undertaken prior to relocation.

Rotator cuff pathology

Supraspinatus problems account for more than a third of all shoulder problems. The subacromial space is just a few millimetres wide and through it passes the biceps tendon, supraspinatus tendon and the subacromial bursa (Figure 28.2).

The 'painful arc' of movement between about 60 and 120° of abduction most commonly results from impingement of the supraspinatus tendon following acute injury and in patients with tendonitis.

Acute tears

This usually involves the supraspinatus tendon near its distal insertion into the greater tuberosity of the humerus. Pain is experienced in the lateral aspect of the upper arm, during abduction and on resisted abduction. It occurs in young active adults after trauma or following a period of impingement and degenerative change in the middle-aged and elderly. Acute tears in the young may warrant surgical repair, otherwise management is conservative with early physiotherapy.

Subacromial bursitis

This typically occurs after periods of unaccustomed exercise in young adults. It presents as dull pain in the anterolateral part of the shoulder at rest, and is another cause of a 'painful arc'.

Calcific tendonitis

This results from calcium deposition in the rotator cuff, particularly near the distal insertion of the supraspinatus tendon. It is typically seen in middle-aged adults, women more than men, and often without evidence of previous rotator cuff pathology.

The condition presents with the sudden onset of severe non-traumatic shoulder pain, limited shoulder movements and disturbed sleep.

X-ray reveals calcium deposits within the rotator cuff. A broad arm sling and nonsteroidal analgesia is the standard treatment, though severe cases may benefit from a steroid injection with local anaesthetic.

Ruptured biceps (long head) and tendonitis

Repeated stresses on the biceps tendon in the subacromial space from repetitive movements of the arm above the head cause inflammation of the biceps and pain on the anterior aspect of the upper arm. This is treated acutely with early mobilisation and nonsteroidal analgesia. Physiotherapy may help in cases that do not settle quickly.

Subsequently, the biceps tendon is prone to degenerative change, which can ultimately result in an acute rupture either spontaneously or after minor trauma. There is sudden pain and a characteristic bulge of the biceps muscle ('Popeye' sign). Treatment is usually conservative, but surgery may be considered in young athletic patients.

Frozen shoulder (adhesive capsulitis)

This can occur after repeated trauma or after any painful condition of the shoulder that results in a restriction of movement. There is an inflammatory reaction within the glenohumeral joint capsule and subsequent adhesions with contraction of the joint capsule.

It is seen typically at ages 40–70, and is more common in diabetics. It characteristically produces an aching night pain with restriction in both active *and* passive movements.

▶ **Diagnoses not to be missed**

Posterior glenohumeral dislocation

Posterior dislocation occurs following a direct blow to the anterior shoulder or a fall onto an internally rotated arm. Posterior dislocations should be suspected in any patient with a painful shoulder following an electrocution or seizure. The shoulder can look near-normal on inspection. The arm is held in adduction and internal rotation and, crucially, there is a gross restriction in movement. There are also subtle X-ray changes on the anterior–posterior view with a symmetrical appearance of the humeral head (the 'light-bulb' sign) and an increased distance to the glenoid rim (the 'rim' sign) (Figure 28.3). The axial/lateral view will usually prove diagnostic.

Radiculopathy

Referred pain from C5–6 disc prolapse can give rise to shoulder pain. It is important to elicit a history of neck problems and pain, and to examine the neck to determine whether certain movements provoke the pain.

Medical conditions

Ischaemic chest pain, diaphragmatic irritation and biliary tree pathology can all give rise to referred pain to the shoulder. These conditions should be considered in any patient where there is poorly localised pain with no clear history of trauma.

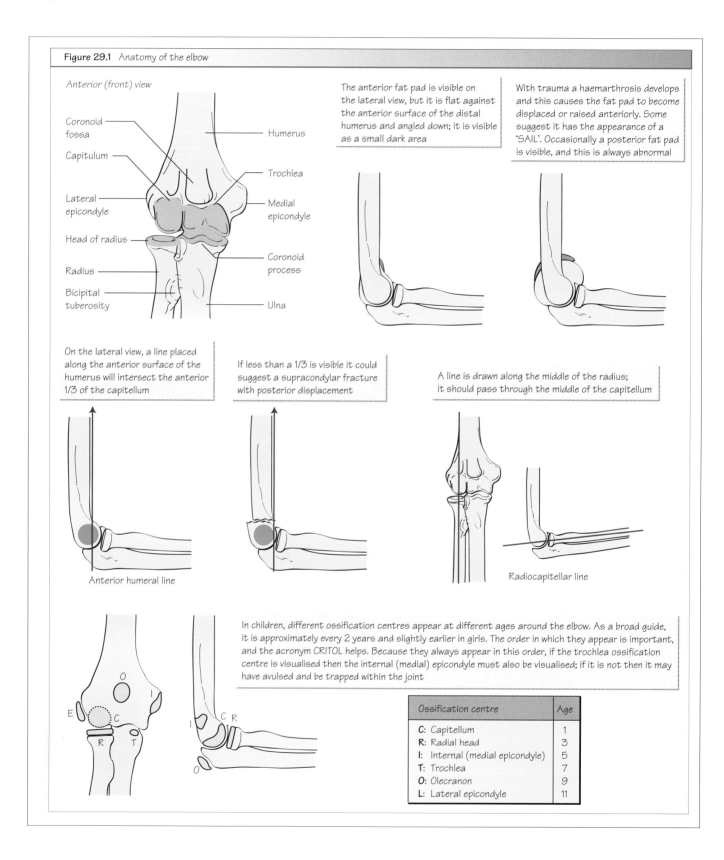

Figure 29.1 Anatomy of the elbow

Anterior (front) view

Coronoid fossa
Capitulum
Lateral epicondyle
Head of radius
Radius
Bicipital tuberosity

Humerus
Trochlea
Medial epicondyle
Coronoid process
Ulna

The anterior fat pad is visible on the lateral view, but it is flat against the anterior surface of the distal humerus and angled down; it is visible as a small dark area

With trauma a haemarthrosis develops and this causes the fat pad to become displaced or raised anteriorly. Some suggest it has the appearance of a 'SAIL'. Occasionally a posterior fat pad is visible, and this is always abnormal

On the lateral view, a line placed along the anterior surface of the humerus will intersect the anterior 1/3 of the capitellum

If less than a 1/3 is visible it could suggest a supracondylar fracture with posterior displacement

A line is drawn along the middle of the radius; it should pass through the middle of the capitellum

Anterior humeral line

Radiocapitellar line

In children, different ossification centres appear at different ages around the elbow. As a broad guide, it is approximately every 2 years and slightly earlier in girls. The order in which they appear is important, and the acronym CRITOL helps. Because they always appear in this order, if the trochlea ossification centre is visualised then the internal (medial) epicondyle must also be visualised; if it is not then it may have avulsed and be trapped within the joint

Ossification centre	Age
C: Capitellum	1
R: Radial head	3
I: Internal (medial epicondyle)	5
T: Trochlea	7
O: Olecranon	9
L: Lateral epicondyle	11

The elbow is classed as a hinge joint. It is capable of flexion and extension, and the superior radio-ulnar joint also allows the forearm to supinate and pronate.

Approach to the patient

In injuries consider whether the force is direct, as in landed on the elbow itself, or indirect, such as falling onto an outstretched hand (FOOSH). Establish the timing and duration of symptoms and any aggravating factors. *Look* for any swelling, bruising, deformities. *Feel* – start at the shoulder and work towards the elbow, establishing if there is any tenderness at the distal humerus. Palpate the medial and lateral epicondyle and the olecranon and ensure that they form an equilateral triangle. Ideally with the elbow flexed, palpate the radial head. Continue distally and establish that there is no tenderness to the forearm or wrist. It is extremely important to assess the radial pulse and the sensory and motor function of the ulna, median and radial nerve. *Move* – assess the range of movement flexion/extension and supination/pronation.

Injuries

Simple bruising is suggested by a history of a minor injury, the lack of bony tenderness, and maintenance of full elbow extension: An inability to fully extend the elbow suggests a haemarthrosis and indicates the need for an X-ray. In an adult this is usually the result of a radial head fracture, and in a child a supracondylar fracture.

Radial head fractures

This is the commonest fracture around the elbow seen in adults and is the result of either direct force or indirect force via a FOOSH. Tenderness over the radial head, lack of full extension and pain on rotation are the usual signs. Some radial head fractures are very subtle and often only the 'fat pad sign' is visible on X-ray. Treatment is with a collar and cuff and orthopaedic follow-up.

Olecranon fractures

These are usually sustained by a fall onto the point of the elbow. Proximal displacement of the fragment is commonly seen as a result of contraction of the triceps. There will be quite marked diffuse swelling and tenderness over the olecranon and the patient will be unable to fully extend. Ensure that the radial head is not dislocated and refer for orthopaedic advice.

Supracondylar fractures

In adults these are often seen in the elderly following a fall and can be a mixture of transverse, oblique and comminuted fracture patterns. Comminuted fractures are often T or Y shaped and involve the articular surface in 95% of cases. The child will have a tender distal humerus and would be unwilling to be examined or move the arm. It is sometimes mistaken as a 'pulled elbow'. It is extremely important to examine and record the distal neurovascular status of the forearm as a fracture can impinge on the brachial artery or median nerve. X-ray appearances can be subtle, but finding a positive fat pad sign in a child is suggestive.

Dislocations

Dislocations of the elbow are relatively common and the deformity is usually obvious. A thorough neurovascular assessment should be documented both pre- and post-reduction.

Pulled elbow

Common in children aged 1–4, following a sudden pull on the arm; for example a child stumbling with the parent pulling hard on the arm to prevent them falling or lifting them up by their arms. Some children are more prone than others and may have had previous episodes. The child presents with the arm hanging limp by their side. The child is often not distressed and appears to be able to play without any discomfort but will clearly not be using the affected arm. There is no pain on palpation, but they will start to cry when attempting to move the elbow. If in any doubt over the history or your clinical findings, X-ray to exclude a supracondylar fracture prior to manipulation. Manipulation is performed by actively supinating the forearm with the elbow flexed whilst palpating the radial head. A click and pain are followed by a return to active movement when successful.

Soft tissue problems

Epicondylitis

Lateral (tennis elbow) is the most common and is characterised by an aching pain that is worsened with activity. The patient may complain of a weak painful grip and have tenderness over the lateral epicondyle and perhaps more distally over the radial head. Resisted extension of the middle finger or wrist with the elbow in extension will reproduce the pain. First-line treatment consists of a short course of anti-inflammatory medication.

Olecranon bursitis

Pain, redness and swelling in the bursa overlying the olecranon process may be the result of a direct blow, or repetitive minor injury due to leaning/rubbing of the elbow against a table. The majority of causes are the result of simple inflammation, but it may be the result of pyogenic infection or gout. Treatment is with nonsteroidal anti-inflammatory drugs and antibiotics for those thought to be infected.

Ulna neuritis/neuropraxia

This is common after a minor blow to the elbow and gives tingling in the ulna nerve distribution. Alternatively, it may be the result of chronic irritation and compression. This typically occurs in middle age and is often associated with diabetes, previous elbow injuries and arthritis.

> ## ► Diagnoses not to be missed
>
> ### Referred pain
>
> Referred pain from the humerus, shoulder and neck can present with elbow symptoms, as can problems with the wrist and distal radial joint.
>
> ### Distal biceps tendon rupture
>
> Usually occurs in middle-aged men or in younger weightlifters. It is characterised by sudden pain over the front of the elbow after a forceful effort against a flexed elbow; for example, lifting something heavy. The patient may hear or feel a snap and develop pain, swelling and bruising around the elbow. Patients will notice loss of strength at the elbow with weakening flexion and supination; for example, turning a door handle or screwdriver. Surgical repair is often indicated.

30 The wrist

Figure 30.1 Bones of the wrist

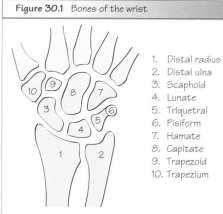

1. Distal radius
2. Distal ulna
3. Scaphoid
4. Lunate
5. Triquetral
6. Pisiform
7. Hamate
8. Capitate
9. Trapezoid
10. Trapezium

Figure 30.2 Checking wrist for (a) flexion and (b) extension

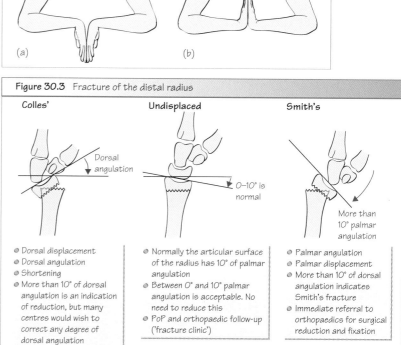

Figure 30.3 Fracture of the distal radius

Colles' — Dorsal angulation

Undisplaced — 0–10° is normal

Smith's — More than 10° palmar angulation

- Dorsal displacement
- Dorsal angulation
- Shortening
- More than 10° of dorsal angulation is an indication of reduction, but many centres would wish to correct any degree of dorsal angulation

- Normally the articular surface of the radius has 10° of palmar angulation
- Between 0° and 10° palmar angulation is acceptable. No need to reduce this
- PoP and orthopaedic follow-up ('fracture clinic')

- Palmar angulation
- Palmar displacement
- More than 10° of dorsal angulation indicates Smith's fracture
- Immediate referral to orthopaedics for surgical reduction and fixation

Figure 30.4 Reduction of a Colles fracture

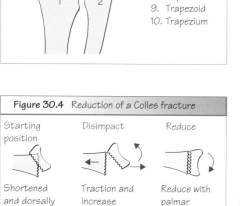

Starting position — Shortened and dorsally angulated

Disimpact — Traction and increase deformity

Reduce — Reduce with palmar angulation and ulnar deviation

Figure 30.5 Finklestein's test (de Quervain's tenosynovitis)

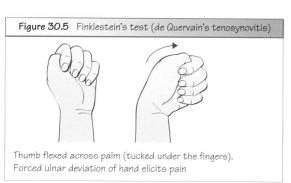

Thumb flexed across palm (tucked under the fingers). Forced ulnar deviation of hand elicits pain

Figure 30.6 Tests for carpal tunnel syndrome. (a) Phalen test, (b) Tinel test

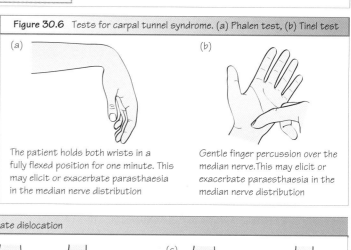

(a) The patient holds both wrists in a fully flexed position for one minute. This may elicit or exacerbate parasthaesia in the median nerve distribution

(b) Gentle finger percussion over the median nerve. This may elicit or exacerbate paraesthaesia in the median nerve distribution

Figure 30.7 (a) Saucer, cup, apple, (b) lunate dislocation, (c) perilunate dislocation

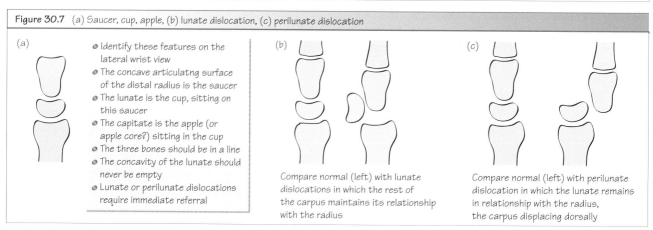

(a)
- Identify these features on the lateral wrist view
- The concave articulatng surface of the distal radius is the saucer
- The lunate is the cup, sitting on this saucer
- The capitate is the apple (or apple core?) sitting in the cup
- The three bones should be in a line
- The concavity of the lunate should never be empty
- Lunate or perilunate dislocations require immediate referral

(b) Compare normal (left) with lunate dislocations in which the rest of the carpus maintains its relationship with the radius

(c) Compare normal (left) with perilunate dislocation in which the lunate remains in relationship with the radius, the carpus displacing dorsally

Minor Injury and Minor Illness at a Glance, First Edition. Edited by Francis Morris, Jim Wardrope, and Shammi Ramlakhan.

Approach to the patient

A brief history should include background details: medical history, medication, allergies, dominant hand and occupation/activities, as well as previous wrist injuries, problems and treatments. *Clarify:* is the problem caused by acute injury, overuse or for no obvious cause? Consider the occupational history, as repetitive load-bearing work, especially at extremes of range of motion, can cause wrist pain. New activities, or sporting equipment with wrong-sized hand-grips, can abnormally load wrist structures. In traumatic injury, a good understanding of the mechanism of injury will clarify your thinking and examination.

Examine the elbow and forearm to exclude injuries, and also the hand. Then examine the wrist itself (Figure 30.1) – remember to examine palmar and dorsal surfaces, and always compare with the other wrist. In particular: **look** for swelling, skin changes, wounds and scars; **feel** the pulses, and test for sensation; **palpate** for bony tenderness, specifically to distal radius and ulna and scaphoid. Palpate the other carpal bones and metacarpals; **move** wrist: flexion and extension (Figure 30.2), pronation and supination.

Injuries

Fractures of the wrist, and soft tissue injuries 'sprains' are common. Mechanism of injury varies, but 'fall onto outstretched hand' is by far the commonest.

Fracture of distal radius and ulna (Figure 30.3)

Minimally displaced fractures of the distal radius and ulna in which there are no neurovascular deficit or skin defect can be treated with simple Plaster of Paris (PoP) backslab and orthopaedic follow-up.

Displaced fractures of the distal radius are common, particularly in the osteoporotic. The fracture fragment of the distal radius typically becomes dorsally displaced, dorsally angulated, radially displaced and impacted, giving rise to the 'dinner fork' deformity.

Local management of these Colles-type injuries may vary, but in the elderly patient this fracture should be reduced (see Figure 30.4) under regional or local block, and immobilised with PoP backslab. More than 10° of dorsal angulation is an indication for reduction. In the younger patient, with high-energy injuries, and those with more complicated fractures, such as Smith's and Barton fractures and compound fractures, orthopaedic assessment is required.

Scaphoid fracture

If there is particular tenderness in the scaphoid region, 'scaphoid views' should be requested. Tenderness in the scaphoid region should be assessed by: palpation of the **anatomical snuff box** – between extensor pollicis longus (EPL) and abductor pollicis longus (APL) and extensor polllicis brevis (EPB); palpation of the **proximal pole of the scaphoid** (palmar surface of wrist); **axial compression** of the thumb metacarpal.

If a scaphoid fracture is seen on X-ray, the wrist should be immobilised in a scaphoid plaster with orthopaedic follow-up.

When scaphoid tenderness is found but X-rays are normal, the wrist should be immobilised with a splint, or a scaphoid plaster, and follow-up arranged within 10–14 days. Asymptomatic patients without persisting tenderness may be discharged at this time. Symptomatic patients require further X-rays and then alternative imaging. Computed tomography/magnetic resonance imaging should be considered if the X-rays still remain normal.

Triquetral fracture

Small bony fragments over the dorsum of the carpus usually indicate triquetral fracture. Treatment: PoP and orthopaedic follow-up ('fracture clinic').

Wrist 'sprain'

Patients with painful wrists following an injury who do not have scaphoid tenderness and normal X-rays are treated as having a soft tissue injury, with a wrist support and analgesia.

Non-traumatic problems

De Quervain's tenosynovitis

This condition is a specific form of tenosynovitis affecting APL and EPB. It is the only commonly encountered tendonitis involving the extensor tendon. Look for pain over these tendons, around the radial styloid and more generally around the radial aspect of the wrist and thumb. Forced ulnar deviation, with the thumb flexed across the palm, may elicit pain (Finklestein test, Figure 30.5).

Management is symptomatic in the first instance, with a wrist and thumb splint and analgesia.

Steroid injections may be helpful and should be offered to patients with persisting symptoms.

Carpal tunnel syndrome

Compression of the median nerve beneath the flexor retinaculum of the wrist gives rise to carpal tunnel syndrome. This condition, which is often bilateral, gives rise to pain, numbness and tingling in the distribution of the median nerve. The pain, which is frequently worse at night, may radiate up the arm to the elbow. The tingling and numbness typically affects the thumb, index, middle and the radial border of the ring finger.

The Phalen test may provoke symptoms, as might the Tinel test (Figure 30.6).

Paratendinitis crepitans

This condition is usually associated with overuse or new activity. There is localised tenderness, swelling and crepitus over the radial dorsal foramen proximal to the wrist. The site of the pain and tenderness is where the radial extensor tendons to the wrist and thumb cross over each other. Treatment is symptomatic with rest, splint and analgesia.

> ▶ **Diagnoses not to be missed**
>
> **Lunate or perilunate dislocation**
>
> Check the lateral view for the apple (capitate), cup (lunate), and saucer (distal radius). (Figure 30.7). They should be in a straight line, and the concavity of the lunate should never be empty. Refer immediately for surgery if lunate/perilunate dislocation is found.
>
> **Pseudogout**
>
> A relatively common condition affecting the wrist, typically in the elderly, is pseudogout. This condition gives rise to a painful swollen red wrist which may appear after minor trauma or spontaneously and may resemble septic arthritis. Patients or their carers are concerned that the wrist may be broken, but the absence of significant trauma, no obvious fracture on the X-ray and calcification of the triangular fibrocartilage allow the diagnosis to be made.

Figure 31.1 Normal cascade

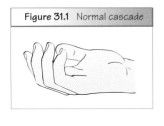

Figure 31.2 Testing FDP

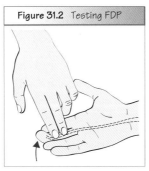

Figure 31.3 Testing FDS

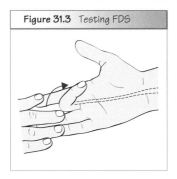

Figure 31.4 Testing extensor indices and extensor digitis minimi

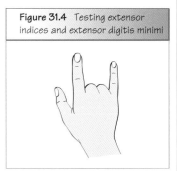

Figure 31.5 Testing the central slip of the extensor mechanism

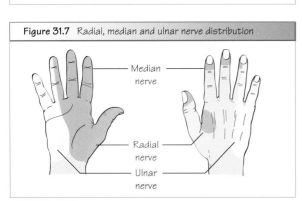

Central slip injury. Attempted active extension at the PIPJ elicits hyper-extension of the distal phalanx

Figure 31.6 Range of movements of the thumb

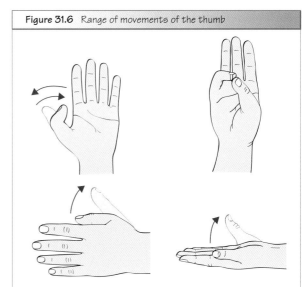

Figure 31.7 Radial, median and ulnar nerve distribution

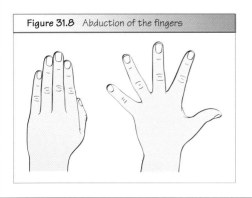

- Median nerve
- Radial nerve
- Ulnar nerve

Figure 31.9 Testing motor function of the ulnar nerve – Froment's sign

When the motor function of the ulnar nerve is damaged, the patient is unable to grasp the paper on removal without flexing their thumb

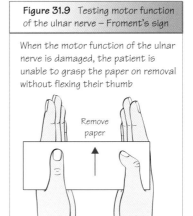

Remove paper

Figure 31.8 Abduction of the fingers

Figure 31.10 Two-point discrimination

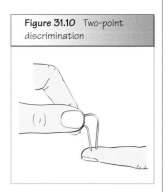

Minor Injury and Minor Illness at a Glance, First Edition. Edited by Francis Morris, Jim Wardrope, and Shammi Ramlakhan.

The hand is a complex structure with many different functions. Injury to the hand or fingers which may appear trivial can give rise to permanent and significant disability and, as a result, may have a significant impact upon the patient both at home and at work. Hand injuries are common, and approximately 30% of them are work-related injuries.

You need a clear understanding of anatomy and how to assess the hand in order to make an accurate diagnosis and offer the patient the appropriate treatment.

Approach to the patient

Stop any bleeding by direct pressure and ensure that the patient has adequate pain relief.

Establish the mechanism of injury; for example, 'bent finger back', crush, punch (against what: mouth/tooth/wall?). The position of the hand or finger at the time of injury is particularly important when assessing for tendon damage. If a wound, was there contamination? Check hand dominance, including any specific functional requirements for hobbies or employment (e.g. piano player). Previous injuries may have left a residual deformity or disability (e.g. nerve damage). A general history should be taken, including the past medical history, medications, allergies and the patient's tetanus status.

Assessment of the hand and fingers

Many patients with painful hand injuries feel faint on examination and it is useful to have the option to lay the patient down if required. Refer to the fingers as index, middle, ring and little (rather than second, third, etc.) and to the volar (palmar), dorsal, back, radial and ulnar surfaces when describing the hand or digits.

• *Look.* The hand should be observed in a relaxed position and the normal cascade of the fingers should be noted (Figure 31.1). Lack of a normal cascade may indicate a tendon injury, whilst rotational deformity may indicate a bone injury. Observe for swelling, deformity, wounds and colour.

• *Feel.* The patient should give an indication as to the most painful point and the clinician should commence their examination away from the site of the injury and work in systematic manner working towards the maximal point of tenderness. The wrist should always be included.

The flexor tendons are assessed with both active and resisted movements. If there is a wound and the tendon is visible, ask the patient to move the finger through the position the hand was in at the time of injury.

Flexor digitorum profundus (FDP) is assessed by asking the patient to flex the distal phalanx whilst immobilising the proximal interphalangeal joint (Figure 31.2).

The flexor digitorum superficialis (FDS) is assessed one finger at a time, by holding the remaining fingers in extension and asking the patient to flex the unrestrained finger (Figure 31.3).

Some patients have a congenital absence of FDS function to the little finger, and this is usually in the dominant hand.

The long extensor tendon (extensor digitorum communis) is assessed by asking the patient to place their hand on the table and lifting each finger individually.

Extensor indices and extensor digitis minimi may be tested in isolation by asking the patient to flex the middle and ring fingers at the *metacarpophalangeal* joints and actively extend the index and little fingers (Figure 31.4).

The central slip of the extensor tendon may be tested by flexing the proximal interphalangeal joint (PIPJ) to 90° over the edge of a table and asking the patient to actively extend the finger against resistance (Figure 31.5). Hypertension at the distal interphalangeal joint is observed when the central slip is damaged (Elson's test).

The range of movements of the thumb should be assessed and the individual tendons flexor and extensor pollicis longus (Figure 31.6).

The nerve supply to the hand should then be assessed. Three nerves supply the hand: radial, median and ulna (Figure 31.7). The motor function of the radial, median and ulna nerves are assessed as follows:

• Radial nerve – dorsiflexion of the wrist against resistance.
• Median nerve – Abduction and opposition of the thumb against resistance.
• Ulnar nerve – Abduction of the fingers against resistance (Figure 31.8) and adduction by asking the patient to cross their fingers. Adduction of the thumb is assessed by asking the patient to grasp a sheet of paper between the thumb and the border of their hand (Figure 31.9). An ability to do this without flexing the thumb, when an attempt to remove the paper is made, indicates that the ulnar nerve is intact.

Sensation is assessed using light touch initially. If there is suspicion of a nerve damage, sharp/blunt or two-point discrimination is used, asking the patient to look away whilst you assess whether they can differentiate between the two (Figure 31.10).

Allen's test is used to assess the patency of the radial and ulnar arteries by compressing both arteries and exanguinating the hand through clenching the fist repeatedly. One artery should be released and the hand should 'pink up' within 3–5 s. This should be repeated testing the other artery. Capillary refill should also be assessed in the digits.

All findings should be documented systematically and concisely.

Figure 32.1 Topographical anticipation: palmar aspect of the hand

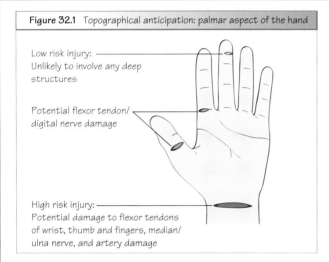

Low risk injury:
Unlikely to involve any deep structures

Potential flexor tendon/digital nerve damage

High risk injury:
Potential damage to flexor tendons of wrist, thumb and fingers, median/ulna nerve, and artery damage

Figure 32.2 Application of paper stitches

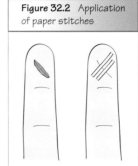

Figure 32.3 Potential bite injuries and damage to the dorsum of the hand and wrist

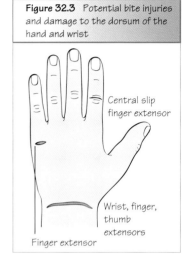

Central slip finger extensor

Wrist, finger, thumb extensors

Finger extensor

Figure 32.4 Drainage of a subungal haematoma

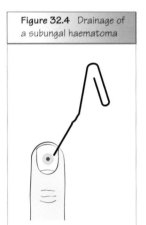

Figure 32.5 Nail bed repair

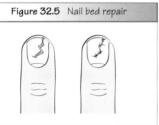

Figure 32.6 Foreign body beneath nail

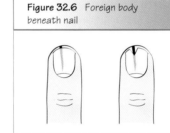

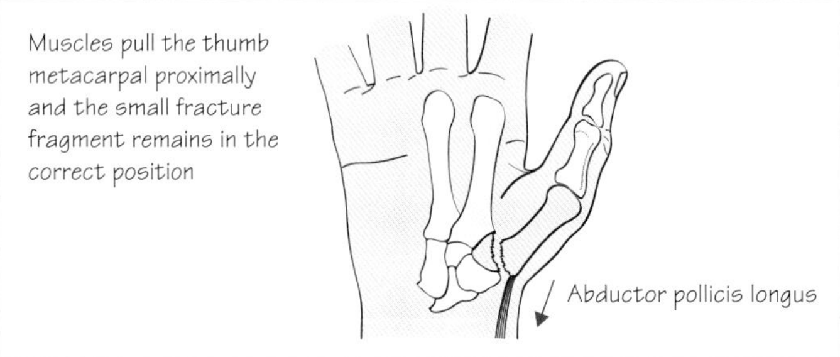

Figure 32.8 Ulnar collateral ligament injury

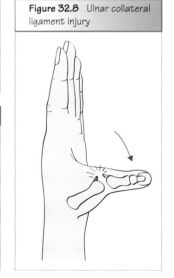

Figure 32.7 Bennett's fracture dislocation

Muscles pull the thumb metacarpal proximally and the small fracture fragment remains in the correct position

Abductor pollicis longus

Minor Injury and Minor Illness at a Glance, First Edition. Edited by Francis Morris, Jim Wardrope, and Shammi Ramlakhan.

General approach to hand wounds

Identify the exact mechanism of injury. Glass and knives often cut to the bone, causing nerve or tendon damage. Wounds from teeth (punch injury), bites and high-pressure grease guns need to be recognised from the outset. All wounds caused by glass require an X-ray to exclude a foreign body (FB), and all rings need to be removed.

Using your knowledge of anatomy – topographical anticipation – ensures that all structures beneath a wound are assessed to confirm that they are functionally intact (Figure 32.1). For example, anticipate digital nerve damage in a patient with clear injury to a digital artery as the two are closely associated.

All wounds need to be cleaned thoroughly; depending upon the type of wound, this can be achieved by using a variety of techniques, such as thorough washing with soap and water through to formal irrigation with saline and exploration using a local anaesthetic. Effective cleaning of wounds is essential to limit wound infections.

Deep, complex wounds, particularly over high-risk areas such as the volar aspect of the wrist and wounds to the metacarpalphalangeal joint (MCPJ) caused by teeth, should be managed by an experienced surgeon.

Adhesive paper strips are useful in closing burst injuries to the finger tips, and sutures are required for wounds that will be under tension. Care should be taken not to apply the paper strips circumferentially as the finger may swell and cause a reduction in blood flow (Figure 32.2). For those patients with wounds without evidence of underlying damage, dress the wound and elevate in a high arm sling, reminding the patient to gently mobilise the hand and fingers. Review all significant wounds at 48 h to ensure tendon and nerve damage has not been overlooked.

Specific wounds
Suspected tendon damage

Resisted movement of tendons should be assessed as up to 90% of the tendon may be severed, but the range of movement preserved. Suspect tendon damage if there is pain on resisted flexion and refer for surgical exploration.

Bites to the hand

Bites to the hand carry a high risk of infection, particular over the MCPJ. This type of injury often occurs when the patient's hand strikes a tooth in a fight (Figure 32.3). These injuries may appear benign but can develop serious complications. If there is bony tenderness or suspicion of an FB, X-ray the wound. The wound should be explored thoroughly for tendon damage and to allow adequate cleaning.

Refer the patient to a hand specialist if there is underlying damage to tendons, bones or the suspicion of joint involvement. Uncomplicated injuries require antibiotics, elevation and a review at 48 h.

The patient should be advised to return if signs of infection (e.g. lymphangitis) or systematic symptoms (e.g. rigors, sweats) develop.

Nail and nail bed injuries

A common injury to the fingertip is a subungal haematoma, usually the result of a crush injury, and is characterised by a throbbing pain and blood under the nail. The blood may be released by drilling a hole through the nail *distal* to the germinal matrix (white half-moon shape) with a white needle (19G), a battery-operated drill or a paper-clip (Figure 32.4). If a fracture is present, prophylactic antibiotics are recommended. If the base of the nail remains in the nail fold, the nail need not be removed to inspect the nail bed, irrespective of the size of the haematoma.

However, nail bed lacerations should be inspected when the nail is dislodged or completely avulsed. Remove the nail from the nail bed with a pair of fine scissors and suture the lacerations with 6/0 vicryl (Figure 32.5). The nail (or suitable replacement) should be cleaned and trimmed and be replaced under the nail fold to allow for new growth of the nail and held in place by paper stitches or a suture.

Foreign bodies

Foreign bodies under the nail (e.g. splinters) are extremely painful. If the FB cannot be removed with splinter forceps, a V-shaped wedge of nail can be removed using local anaesthetic to allow access (Figure 32.6).

Thermal injuries (see Chapter 6)

For patients with a thermal injury consisting of simple erythema the hand should be rinsed with cool tap water and a petroleum-based dressing should be applied.

Partial-thickness burns are treated by applying a silver-based cream to prevent infection either on a sterile dressing or in a 'hand bag' to allow full movement of the fingers. Special consideration should be given to hand and finger function during the healing process, and all significant and full-thickness hand burns require specialist assessment.

Thumb injuries

A Bennett's fracture is an oblique intra-articular fracture of the base of the metacarpal to the thumb associated with radial subluxation of the metacarpal itself. Muscles to the thumb pull the metacarpal proximally whilst the fragment of bone remains in place (Figure 32.7). It is often caused when the thumb is hyperextended or 'bent backwards' and is a common skiing injury. This type of injury should be referred to the hand specialist.

Non-displaced fractures of the proximal and distal phalanges to the thumb may be followed up in the fracture clinic.

A very common injury to the thumb is a sprain to the MCPJ which involves the collateral ligaments, usually the ulnar (Figure 32.8). There is often a history of hyperextension or abduction, and X-rays may reveal an avulsion fracture from the base of the proximal phalanx. On assessment, the stability of the ulna collateral ligament needs to be assessed as lax ligaments require referral to a hand specialist.

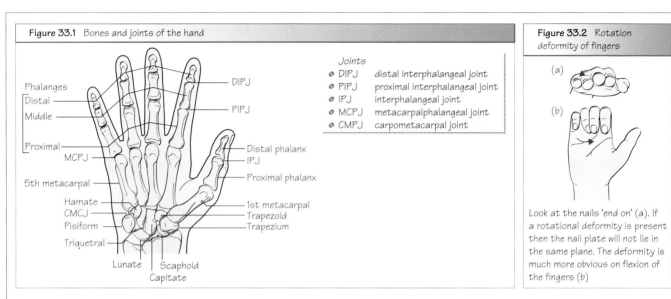

Figure 33.1 Bones and joints of the hand

Phalanges
Distal
Middle
Proximal
MCPJ
5th metacarpal
Hamate
CMCJ
Pisiform
Triquetral
Lunate
Scaphoid
Capitate

DIPJ
PIPJ
Distal phalanx
IPJ
Proximal phalanx
1st metacarpal
Trapezoid
Trapezium

Joints
- DIPJ   distal interphalangeal joint
- PIPJ   proximal interphalangeal joint
- IPJ   interphalangeal joint
- MCPJ   metacarpalphalangeal joint
- CMPJ   carpometacarpal joint

Figure 33.2 Rotation deformity of fingers

(a)

(b)

Look at the nails 'end on' (a). If a rotational deformity is present then the nail plate will not lie in the same plane. The deformity is much more obvious on flexion of the fingers (b)

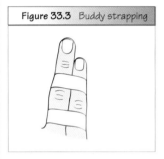

Figure 33.3 Buddy strapping

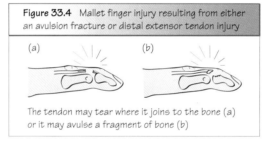

Figure 33.4 Mallet finger injury resulting from either an avulsion fracture or distal extensor tendon injury

(a)   (b)

The tendon may tear where it joins to the bone (a) or it may avulse a fragment of bone (b)

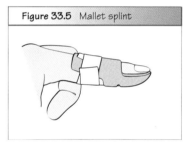

Figure 33.5 Mallet splint

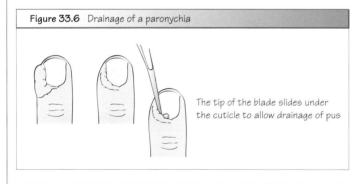

Figure 33.6 Drainage of a paronychia

The tip of the blade slides under the cuticle to allow drainage of pus

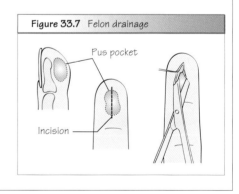

Figure 33.7 Felon drainage

Pus pocket

Incision

Minor Injury and Minor Illness at a Glance, First Edition. Edited by Francis Morris, Jim Wardrope, and Shammi Ramlakhan.

The bones and joints of the hand are shown in Figure 33.1.

Metacarpal fractures

Metacarpal fractures are often caused by a 'punch'-type injury, and some patients are reluctant to admit to how they sustained the injury.

Fifth metacarpal fractures are very common, and closed injuries with minimal displacement can be treated conservatively without patient follow-up.

Refer on to a hand specialist those fractures with the following: rotational deformity (Figure 33.2), volar angulation/unable to extend MCPJ to 0°, compound fractures, multiple metacarpals involved and those with significant displacement.

If a fracture of the base of a metacarpal is suspected, a true lateral should be requested as subluxations and dislocations can be difficult to assess on an oblique X-ray.

Finger fractures

Fractures to the distal phalanx require splintage only. Fractures proximal to the waist of the terminal phalanx or intra-articular fractures of over 25% of the joint surface require referral to a hand specialist for possible stabilisation. Open fractures require prophylactic antibiotic cover to prevent infection.

Dislocations

Dislocations of the finger at the PIPJ and DIPJ are common. The presence of wounds should be noted and the finger X-rayed. A digital nerve block at the level of the metacarpal head should be given and longitudinal traction applied. If there is resistance then a relocation is not achieved; soft tissue interposition should be considered and a referral to a hand specialist made for open reduction. Following successful reduction, a good range of movement should be possible and the finger splinted with buddy strapping (Figure 33.3). The patient should be encouraged to mobilise the finger to prevent long term stiffness and reviewed.

Amputations

Soft tissue injuries to the finger tips that involve skin loss may be managed conservatively if the bone is not exposed and the tissue loss limited. The wound should be thoroughly cleaned under a local anaesthetic ring block, devitalised tissue should be trimmed and a non-adherent, petroleum-based dressing applied, and the patient reviewed after 48 h.

Refer to a hand specialist those patients with finger tip injuries with skin loss ≥1 cm^2 or bone exposure. More significant amputations of the finger will all require referral to a hand specialist.

Care of an amputated finger part: foreign material should be removed and the finger part cleaned with normal saline, then wrapped in a saline-dampened gauze and placed in a plastic bag. The plastic bag should then be placed in a saline and ice-filled container.

Mallet finger

Mallet deformity is caused by the avulsion of the insertion of the extensor tendon into the distal phalanx, usually by forced flexion (Figure 33.4). If left untreated, the patient will be left with a 'hook'-type deformity. Open injuries and those involving a significantly sized avulsion fragment of bone should be referred for formal repair. Otherwise, treat conservatively with a mallet splint, splinting the DIPJ in extension, leaving the PIPJ free movement for 6 weeks (Figure 33.5). Patient compliance is key to a successful outcome, and regular review is required.

Collateral ligament injuries

Sprains of the PIPJ and DIPJ may be treated with a Bedford splint/buddy strapping and the patient asked to mobilise their fingers. Hyperextension injuries to the PIPJs may also involve the volar plate. Volar plate injuries are identified by a tell-tale avulsion flake of bone from the volar margin of the middle phalanx. Patients should be treated with buddy strapping and reviewed as hand physiotherapy may be required.

Other conditions
Paronychia

This is a common infection of the nail fold. Early infections without pus may settle with antibiotics and warm soaks. When pus has collected that is either self-evident on inspection or suspected because of throbbing pain that disturbs the patient's sleep and is worse on dependency, surgical drainage is required. It should be drained by elevating the nail fold, irrigating and packing the cavity (Figure 33.6). Once drained, in the absence of ascending lymphangitis, antibiotics are not required.

Felon

This is a deep-seated infection of the finger pulp, usually following a wound. The patient presents with throbbing, swelling and pain to the distal end of the finger. An X-ray should be taken to exclude osteomyelitis and the infection drained by an experienced surgeon (Figure 33.7).

Arthritis

Osteoarthritis at the base of the thumb is a common cause of pain and disability, and symptoms may be precipitated by minor trauma. X-rays reveal typical changes of sclerosis and osteophytes.

Gout and pseudogout may present with an acutely painful joint in the hands. Affected joints are typically red, painful and swollen and may be associated with tophi. Gout is treated with elevation and splintage, nonsteroidal anti-inflammatory drugs or colchicine and the discontinuation of precipitating drugs such as diuretics. In the absence of penetrating wounds septic arthritis is unusual in the small joints of the hand.

Trigger finger

Trigger finger (or thumb) occurs most commonly with the flexor tendon of the middle and ring fingers and is caused by thickening of the tendon and/or the sheath at the point where the tendon enters the sheath. Patients complain of a locking, catching, clicking or jumping of the affected finger or thumb. There is tenderness at the proximal tendon sheath at the level of the metacarpal head on the palmar aspect of the hand and sometimes a nodule may be felt. Treatment is by injection of steroids into the tendon sheath.

> ### ▶ Diagnoses not to be missed
>
> #### Flexor tendon sheath infection
>
> This usually occurs following a puncture wound and is characterised by the finger held in slight flexion with swelling and pain along the course of the flexor tendon with pain on passive extension of the finger. The patient should be referred for incision, drainage and irrigation of the sheath.

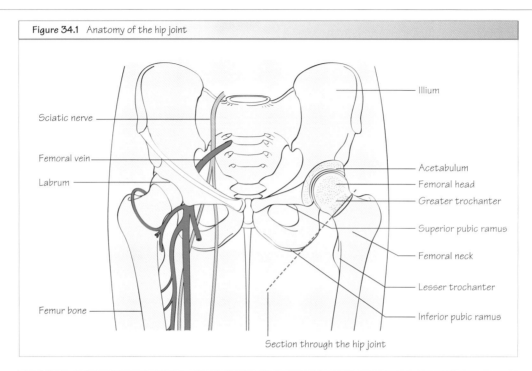

Figure 34.1 Anatomy of the hip joint

Sciatic nerve

Femoral vein

Labrum

Femur bone

Illium

Acetabulum

Femoral head

Greater trochanter

Superior pubic ramus

Femoral neck

Lesser trochanter

Inferior pubic ramus

Section through the hip joint

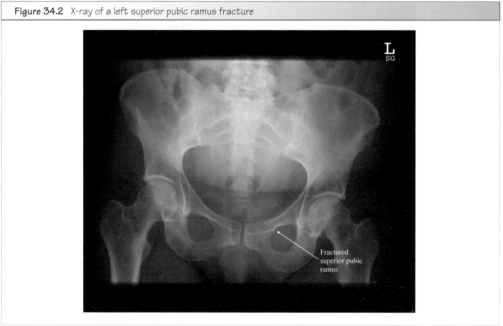

Figure 34.2 X-ray of a left superior pubic ramus fracture

Fractured superior pubic ramus

Minor Injury and Minor Illness at a Glance, First Edition. Edited by Francis Morris, Jim Wardrope, and Shammi Ramlakhan.

The hip joint attaches the leg to the torso and comprises the head of the femur (the ball) that swivels in the acetabulum (the socket), which is made up of the pelvic bones (Figure 34.1).

Approach to the patient

Start with a careful history and identify the nature, mode of onset, associated features and duration of the problem. Many causes of hip pain are related to the joint itself and surrounding muscles, but pain from remote sources can be referred to the hip area. For instance, back and sacroiliac problems may refer to the hip, as may ovarian, vascular (e.g. ruptured aorta) and abdominal pathology.

The examination should include an assessment of the joint above, the spine and sacroiliac joints and the joint below the knee, along with an assessment of the neurovascular supply to the leg, the hernial orifices, external genitalia and the abdomen.
• *Look* for obvious abnormalities, such as rotational deformity, erythema, scars and quadraceps wasting.
• *Feel* for temperature difference and palpate for tenderness over the adductor longus tendon, greater trochanter, ischial tuberosity, sacroiliac joint and low back.
• *Move (actively and passively).*
• *Special tests.* Thomas's test. The test checks for a fixed flexion deformity. Ask the patient to lie flat with your hand under the lower part of their back to remove any lumbar lordosis. In turn, flex each leg fully to see if the other leg remains flat. If it does not this may indicate a fixed flexion of that hip.

If possible, then assess the patient's gait.

Injuries

Simple falls in the elderly are a common cause of fractures around the hip. These range from pubic rami fractures (Figure 34.2) that need symptomatic treatment to neck of femur fractures which need surgery. Impacted fractures of the femoral neck may occur after relatively trivial trauma, and the patient may still be able to mobilise. X-rays are indicated in any patient over 55 with new onset of hip pain following a fall. Likewise, X-rays are indicated in any patient who cannot weight bear following a fall whatever the age. If the X-ray is normal and the patient still very symptomatic magnetic resonance imaging (MRI) is indicated.

In the relatively young, repeated high-impact activities and overuse can result in a stress fracture of the hip. A stress fracture is a break in the bone that occurs when minor injuries to the bone build up beyond the capacity of the bone to repair itself. Stress fractures of the hip are recognised in runners and can be difficult to diagnose. Typical symptoms include gradual onset of poorly localised pain provoked by exercise. X-rays may be diagnostic if the symptoms have been present for a number of weeks, otherwise computed tomography or MRI is required.

A pelvic avulsion fracture is caused by a strong muscular contraction pulling a fragment of bone away from its attachment point. This occurs in adolescents who are athletic and most commonly involves the ischial tuberosity where the hamstrings attach. Tenderness will be present and symptoms provoked by passive stretch or resisted contraction of the muscle involved. An X-ray will confirm the diagnosis. Treatment will usually be the same as for soft tissue injuries and will usually be symptomatic.

Soft tissue injuries

Muscular strains around the hip and groin are common, especially in sports people. Adductor muscle strains are common and present with acute onset of pain during exercise and are frequently the result of a sudden change in direction.

The pain is well localised on the inner aspect of the upper thigh either in the belly of the adductor longus or near its origin on the pubic rami.

Passive abduction and resisted adduction reproduce the symptoms. Treatment is symptomatic.

Non-traumatic problems
Osteoarthritis

Wear and tear of the hip joint is extremely common in the middle-aged and elderly. Pain on walking and stiffness are common symptoms, and hip joint movements are typically restricted with loss of internal rotation and extension. Acute exacerbations may be provoked by minor trauma, loose bodies, and so on, though serious complications such as sepsis may need excluding.

Septic arthritis

Septic arthritis of the hip joint must be considered in a patient presenting with non-traumatic hip pain with systemic upset. This is especially the case if the patient is immunocompromised or has a prosthetic joint. Patients where this diagnosis is likely need urgent referral to the orthopaedic team for consideration of joint aspiration/washout. A delay in management may lead to damage to the joint and higher rates of morbidity and mortality.

Trochanteric bursitis

This is a common problem that causes inflammation and tenderness in the bursa over the lateral thigh. Acute or repetitive trauma may give rise to inflammation of the bursa between the femoral trochanteric process and the gluteus medius/iliotibial tract. Point tenderness is found over the greater trochanter, and flexion of the hip with adduction provokes the symptoms. Treatment is symptomatic with analgesia and stretching exercises.

► Diagnoses not to be missed

Femoral hernia

Always ensure that the hernial orifices are assessed, particularly in the elderly.

Referred pain from back

Pain from acute crush fractures of the lumbar spine, degenerative disc disease and nerve root compression can all be experienced in the hip and buttock rather than the back.

---

35 Knee examination

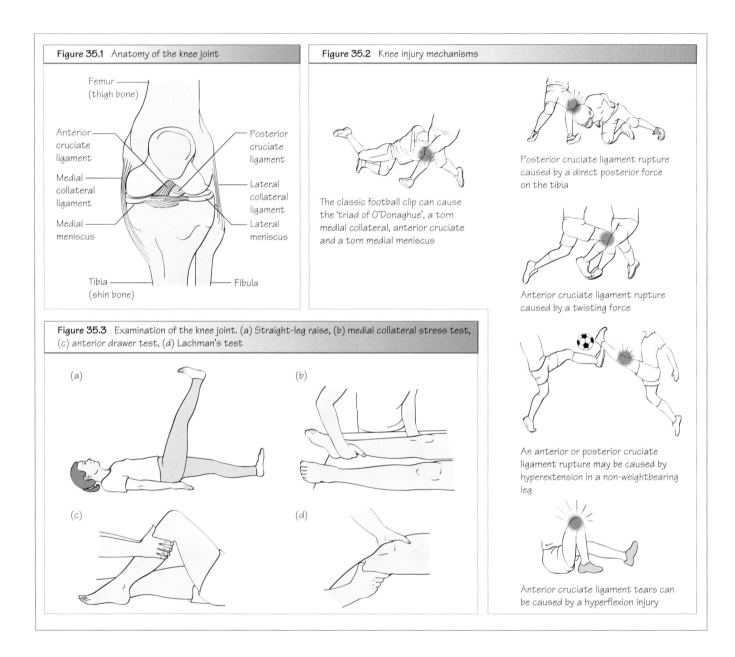

Figure 35.1 Anatomy of the knee joint

Femur (thigh bone)

Anterior cruciate ligament

Medial collateral ligament

Medial meniscus

Tibia (shin bone)

Posterior cruciate ligament

Lateral collateral ligament

Lateral meniscus

Fibula

Figure 35.2 Knee injury mechanisms

The classic football clip can cause the 'triad of O'Donaghue', a torn medial collateral, anterior cruciate and a torn medial meniscus

Posterior cruciate ligament rupture caused by a direct posterior force on the tibia

Anterior cruciate ligament rupture caused by a twisting force

An anterior or posterior cruciate ligament rupture may be caused by hyperextension in a non-weightbearing leg

Anterior cruciate ligament tears can be caused by a hyperflexion injury

Figure 35.3 Examination of the knee joint. (a) Straight-leg raise, (b) medial collateral stress test, (c) anterior drawer test, (d) Lachman's test

(a)

(b)

(c)

(d)

Minor Injury and Minor Illness at a Glance, First Edition. Edited by Francis Morris, Jim Wardrope, and Shammi Ramlakhan.

The knee joint is a complex joint. Its main function is to flex and extend to aid walking. It also twists and rotates. The patella femoral joint is especially important going up and down stairs. The knee relies on a number of structures, including bones, ligaments, tendons and cartilage. Each part of the anatomy needs to function properly for the knee to work (Figure 35.1).

Approach to the patient

The most important aspect of assessing these patients is a detailed history, including the mechanism of injury (Figure 35.2), followed by examination.

While direct blows to the knee occur, the knee is more susceptible to twisting or stretching injuries, as is common in sports, taking the joint through a greater range of motion than it can tolerate.

If the knee is stressed from a specific direction, then the ligament trying to hold it in place against that force can tear. Twisting injuries to the knee put stress on the meniscus and can pinch it between the tibial surface and the edges of the femoral condyle, causing tears.

Injuries of the muscles and tendons surrounding the knee are caused by acute hyperflexion or hyperextension of the knee or by overuse. These strains can result in complete tears at their worst.

Acute knee injuries can cause pain and swelling and difficulty bending the knee and weight-bearing. If the swelling occurs immediately it is strongly suggestive of bleeding within the joint – an acute haemarthrosis. To bleed the damaged structure needs to be vascular; for example, ligaments or bone. The differential diagnosis of a haemarthrosis in a patient without a fracture on X-rays includes ligament damage, patella dislocation, osteochondral injuries and capsular tears. An acute haemarthrosis will always require orthopaedic review. If the swelling arises over a period of many hours, meniscal injuries or a reactive effusion may be the cause.

Pain can sometimes be felt with specific activities. Pain while climbing stairs is a symptom of meniscus injury, where the meniscus is being pinched in the joint as it narrows with bending. Pain with walking down stairs suggests patellar pain, where the kneecap is being forced onto the femur. Giving way, or grinding in the knee, is associated with cartilage or meniscus tears. 'Locking' is the term used when the knee joint refuses to completely straighten, and this is almost always due to torn meniscus. In this situation, the torn piece of meniscus folds upon itself and does not allow the knee to extend.

Anyone unable to weight-bear after a knee injury or who has a history consistent with haemarthrosis requires X-rays looking for fractures, lipo-haemarthrosis, mal-alignment or pre-existing conditions such as osteoarthritis

General approach to examination

Always examine the hip, but especially where there are no signs on knee examination. Note any systemic signs such as a temperature. Injuries can be difficult to assess due to pain, so analgesia should be offered.

Look
- Assess gait prior to laying the patient down.
- Look for:
  - swelling/loss of knee dimple
  - erythema
  - scars
  - quadriceps wasting.

Feel
- Temperature difference.
- Signs of effusion:
  - *Patella tap.* Squeeze fluid out of the supra-patella pouch with one hand and with the other press on the patella. A palpable 'tap' is a positive test.
  - *Fluid displacement.* Squeeze fluid out of the supra-patella pouch, stroke the lateral side and look for distension of the medial side.
- Palpate the following for tenderness: joint line/medial and lateral collaterals/patella/fibula head/tibial tubercle/distal femur.

Move (actively and passively)
- The normal range of motion is from 0° to 135°.
- *Extensor apparatus.* Ask the patient to lift their straightened leg off the bed (straight-leg raise; Figure 35.3a). They may be unable to because of pain, quadriceps rupture, patella fracture or patella ligament rupture, or painful acute haemarthrosis.

Special tests
- *Medial and lateral collateral stress (Figure 35.3b).* With one hand stabilising the upper thigh with the knee flexed at 20°, the lower leg is pushed laterally and then medially to test the laxity of each ligament respectively.
- *Anterior and posterior drawer tests (Figure 35.3c).* With the knee flexed to 90° and the foot stable the lower leg is grabbed firmly with both hands and is first pulled forward and then backward to test the integrity of each respectively.
- *Lachman's test (Figure 35.3d).* One hand secures the distal femur while the other firmly grasps the proximal tibia. A gentle anterior translation force is applied to the proximal tibia. The examiner assesses for anterior translocation of the tibia and anterior cruciate.

Figure 36.1 Knee injuries. (a) Patella fracture, (b) tibial plateau fracture

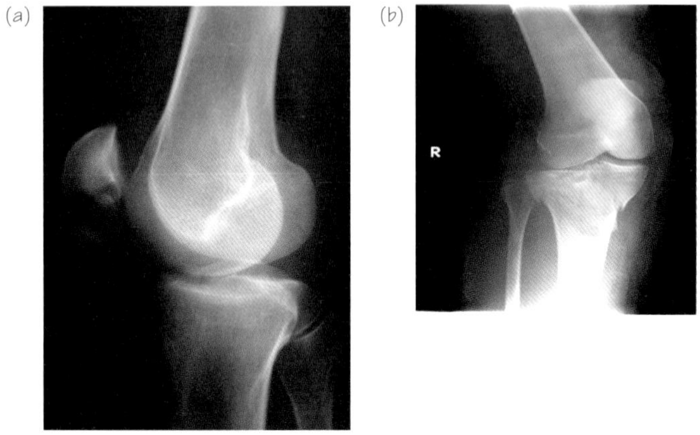

(a)

(b)

R

Figure 36.2 Knee aspiration

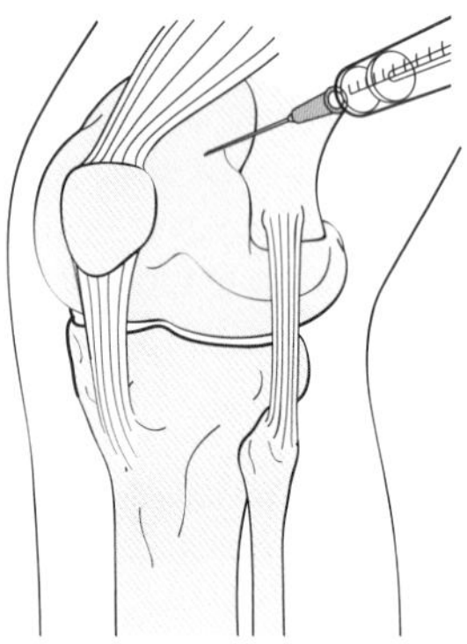

- Ensure full asepsis
- Do not inject through cellulitic area
- Inject local anaesthetic 1 cm above and lateral to patella down to synovium
- Ensure local anaesthetic effective
- Aspirate the joint
- Squeeze sides of joint to empty before removing needle
- Apply sterile dressing
- Note nature of aspirate (blood/pus?)
- Send aspirate for urgent microscopy – cells and crystals
- Await culture and sensitivity
- If septic, refer to orthopaedics
- In the immunosuppressed or those with a prosthesis this should be done in a sterile environment under the orthopaedic surgeons

Figure 36.3 Pathophysiology of septic arthritis. How organisms may invade the joint

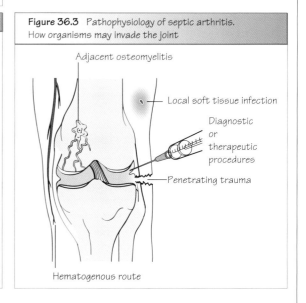

Adjacent osteomyelitis

Local soft tissue infection

Diagnostic or therapeutic procedures

Penetrating trauma

Hematogenous route

Minor Injury and Minor Illness at a Glance, First Edition. Edited by Francis Morris, Jim Wardrope, and Shammi Ramlakhan.

Knee complaints may be classified into traumatic or non-traumatic. Of the traumatic conditions, ligament injuries are common and fractures less so. In this chapter some of the commoner conditions under these categories and their management will be considered.

Traumatic knee problems
Soft tissue injuries
Medial collateral ligament injury
This is a very common sporting injury and results from a valgus stress on the knee. Severity ranges from mild sprains where the patient is able to weight-bear to more severe injury where they are not. On examination there is not usually an effusion as this structure is extra-articular. There will be tenderness over the ligament and increased laxity and/or pain on stressing it. Treatment for the milder picture is symptomatic. For more severe injuries crutches may be necessary as well as follow-up.

Lateral collateral ligament injury
This is a rarer injury. It results from a varus stress on the joint. Again, joint swelling is usually absent and there is localised tenderness over the ligament. Increased laxity on varus testing may be demonstrated. Some patients will have an associated peroneal nerve palsy, so remember to test for dorsiflexion and eversion of the foot and sensory loss. Immediate specialist assessment is required for those with a nerve palsy.

Acute haemarthrosis
A patient with a traumatic haemarthrosis should be considered as having a cruciate ligament injury until proven otherwise. All such patients require orthopaedic follow-up.

Anterior cruciate ligament rupture
This is a common sporting injury and is usually caused by twisting associated with a change in direction. The patient will often hear a 'pop' at the time. Pain is immediate, as is swelling (haemarthrosis). Special tests for this injury may be difficult to perform owing to pain. All patients with suspected haemarthrosis need an X-ray as there may be a lateral capsule or tibial spine avulsion present. Management is symptomatic and the patient should be followed up as an outpatient.

Posterior cruciate ligament rupture
This injury occurs after a direct force on the anterior tibia, such as a dashboard injury or a fall on the flexed knee. Symptoms are similar to those with anterior cruciate damage. There may be posterior sag of the tibia. An X-ray may show subluxation of the tibia or associated fractures. Treatment is symptomatic, and follow-up as an out patient is required.

Meniscal injuries
These are usually due to pivoting forces. Pain and tenderness may be localised, either in the medial or lateral joint lines. The knee may 'lock' and the patient may be unable to straighten it. The patient will have pain on gentle tibial rotation. If the knee is locked a referral to orthopaedics should be made; if not, an outpatient appointment should be made.

Patella tendon/quadriceps tendon rupture
Usually these are due to strong opposed quadriceps contraction; for example a slip with sudden quadriceps contraction. There is immediate pain and swelling and an inability to actively extend the knee. The patient will be unable to straight-leg raise and may have a palpable gap above or below the patella. An X-ray of the knee may show a high-riding (patella tendon rupture) or low-riding (quadriceps tendon rupture) patella. If the diagnosis is in doubt the patient may need an ultrasound or magnetic resonance imaging scan. Immediate repair should be considered.

Fractures
The patella may fracture due to a dashboard injury or a fall directly onto it (Figure 36.1a). This injury will require orthopaedic assessment.

The head of the fibula on the lateral side of the knee joint can be fractured by a direct blow and may be associated with a peroneal nerve palsy. The peroneal nerve wraps around the bone and can be damaged, giving rise to a foot drop.

With jumping injuries, the surface of the tibia can be damaged, resulting in a fracture to the tibial plateau (Figure 36.1b). After X-rays reveal this fracture, a computed tomography scan is usually done to make certain that there is no displacement of the bones. This type of fracture requires an orthopaedic referral.

Non-traumatic knee problems
Crystal arthropathy
Gout and pseudogout are the two most common crystal-induced arthropathies. They are debilitating illnesses in which recurrent episodes of pain and joint inflammation are caused by the formation of crystals within the joint space and deposition of crystals in soft tissue. The knee is a commonly affected joint. Gout is inflammation caused by monosodium urate monohydrate crystals. Pseudogout is inflammation caused by calcium pyrophosphate crystals. An important differential of these conditions is septic arthritis (see 'Diagnoses not to be missed') as all three conditions may give rise to a red-hot painful knee and systemic symptoms. Joint aspiration (Figure 36.2) is an important investigation to differentiate between these conditions. In proven crystal arthropathy, rest and nonsteroidal anti-inflammatory drugs (or colchicine) are the mainstay of initial treatment.

Prepatellar bursitis (housemaid's knee)
The prepatellar bursa is most commonly affected in this condition due to its exposure while kneeling. On examination you may find a warm, fluctuant swelling anterior to the patella, and unlike in septic arthritis the range of motion of the knee is usually preserved. The mainstay of treatment is ice, elevation and anti-inflammatories. In severe cases aspiration and or antibiotics may be necessary.

> ### ▶ Diagnoses not to be missed
>
> #### Referred pain to the knee
>
> Pain from the hip may be referred to the knee. Hip pathology may be felt exclusively in the lower thigh and knee area and is a trap for the unwary. Always examine the hip in a patient with knee symptoms.
>
> #### Septic arthritis
>
> Septic arthritis may represent a direct invasion of joint space by various microorganisms, usually the streptococcus or staphylococcus (Figure 36.3). Failure to recognise and to appropriately treat septic arthritis results in significant rates of morbidity, joint destruction and may even lead to death. Increasing use of prosthetic joints has led to an increased incidence of septic arthritis in the knee.

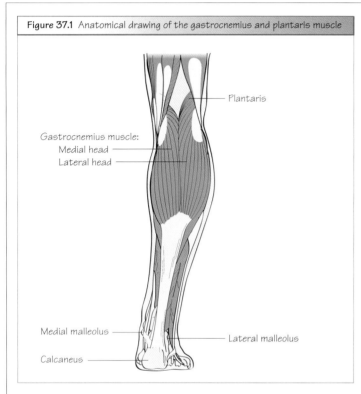

Figure 37.1 Anatomical drawing of the gastrocnemius and plantaris muscle

Plantaris

Gastrocnemius muscle:
Medial head
Lateral head

Medial malleolus

Lateral malleolus

Calcaneus

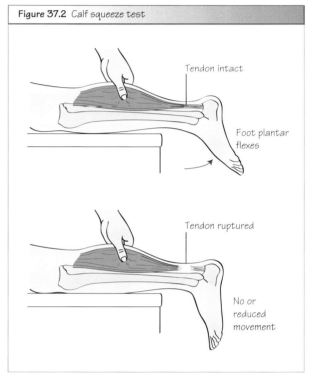

Figure 37.2 Calf squeeze test

Tendon intact

Foot plantar flexes

Tendon ruptured

No or reduced movement

Minor Injury and Minor Illness at a Glance, First Edition. Edited by Francis Morris, Jim Wardrope, and Shammi Ramlakhan.

Approach to patient

Soft tissue injuries to the shin and calf, such as bruising, pretibial lacerations and haematomas, are common and frequently the result of sporting activities, falls and direct blows.

Isolated fractures of the fibula are usually the result of a direct blow and identified by the presence of bony tenderness.

Always examine the knee, ankle, Achilles tendon and confirm peripheral neurovascular integrity when assessing the calf and shin.

Calf muscle injury

A common problem giving rise to sudden acute pain in the calf is a tear of the medial head of the gastrocnemius muscle (Figure 37.1). This injury is commoner in men, typically occurring in individuals who are unaccustomed to regular exercise. The damage occurs when the leg is loaded and the patient is involved in activities such as running up an incline, jumping or suddenly pushing off, as in running (badminton leg). An audible pop or tearing sensation may be felt in the upper medial aspect of the calf associated with sudden pain and limping.

Clinical examination reveals localised tenderness to the medial head of the gastrocnemius muscle which may be associated with some swelling. Bruising and discolouration tends to appear days later when it has a tendency to track down the leg to the ankle.

Treatment consists of advice, analgesia and gentle mobilisation with the aid of crutches and physiotherapy as required.

► Achilles tendon rupture

Partial or complete rupture of the Achilles tendon usually occurs suddenly and the patient may believe they have been struck from behind by an object or kicked. The usual site of the Achilles tendon rupture is approximately 6 cm above its insertion into the calcaneus and, therefore, the site of pain is quite distinct from that of a calf muscle injury.

In a typical case there will be a palpable gap in the Achilles tendon associated with swelling. Rupture is confirmed clinically by performing the calf squeeze test (see Figure 37.2). When positive, squeezing the calf fails to produce plantar flexion movements at the ankle when compared with the normal side.

The patient will still have the ability to actively plantar flex their foot owing to the presence of other intact tendons, such as tibialis posterior and flexor hallucis longus, although plantar flexion will be weak.

Partial ruptures still cause pain, but the calf squeeze test may show intact plantar flexion. Ultrasound is the best way of confirming the diagnosis if partial or complete rupture is suspected.

Treatment choices consist of either conservative immobilisation in plaster or surgical repair.

Ruptured Baker's cyst

A Baker's cyst is an out-pouching of the synovium of the knee joint which occurs in people with inflammatory or degenerative arthritis and gives rise to a fullness in the popliteal fossa. When the fluids leaks out of the synovium into the calf muscle it excites an intense inflammatory response giving rise to the sudden onset of pain and swelling. The moment of rupture may be felt as a sharp pain behind the knee while the patient is engaged in activity that increases the pressure within the joint (e.g. squatting). Alternatively, the leak may occur more insidiously and resemble the onset of a deep venous thrombosis.

Follow-up care for patients with symptomatic Baker's cysts is with their general practitioner.

Thrombophlebitis

Discrete tenderness and thread like lumpiness overlying a superficial vein may give rise to the complaint of calf pain. Superficial thrombophlebitis in the absence of varicose veins is a risk factor for deep venous thrombosis. Treatment, once a deep venous thrombosis has been excluded, is usually symptomatic (analgesia, stockings), while extensive or progressive disease may require low molecular weight heparin.

Deep venous thrombosis

The signs and symptoms of deep venous thrombosis are related to the degree of obstruction and inflammation of the veins involved. In contrast to calf muscle injuries, the onset is usually insidious with aching, tenderness and swelling developing over a number of days or weeks.

Many of the signs are nonspecific, but oedema of the affected leg is one of the most constant findings.

Redness and warmth may be present over the area of thrombosis, and as a result the differential diagnosis of a deep venous thrombosis frequently involves cellulitis. Deep venous thrombosis is slightly more common in men and individuals over the age of 40.

Factors that promote venous stasis, vessel wall injury or are prothrombotic (Virchow's triad) render individuals susceptible to the development of deep venous thrombosis. Examples include prolonged immobility, major surgery and thrombophilias.

Using the Wells risk scoring system and judicious use of the d-dimer blood test helps stratify risk in deciding which patients should undergo further investigation. The diagnosis is confirmed by ultrasonography and treatment consists of anticoagulation with warfarin.

Cellulitis

Cellulitis is common in the lower legs and gives rise to red, tender, painful shins and calves. It is frequently the result of bacteria gaining access through minor breaks in the skin of the shin and foot, especially between the toes. The responsible bacteria are usually staphylococcus or streptococcus. Uncomplicated cases are treated with oral antibiotics.

Vulnerable individuals with diabetes or peripheral vascular disease or those patients who are constitutionally unwell with rigors/vomiting, may require intravenous therapy.

► Diagnoses not to be missed

Achilles tendon rupture

See red flag section in this chapter.

Compartment syndrome

This syndrome, which is characterised by severe and unremitting pain, is usually the result of severe crush injuries, but may occur after relatively minor injuries (e.g. soft tissue bruising), particularly if the patient has a bleeding problem. Disproportionate pain, a tense swollen compartment, an inability to walk and pain on passive stretch of the muscles involved would strongly suggest the diagnosis. Referral for immediate decompression is required.

Arterial insufficiency

Acute arterial insufficiency will result in rest pain involving the whole lower leg and foot associated with pallor, parasthesiae, loss of function (paralysis) and absent pulses.

Figure 38.1 Anatomy of the ankle

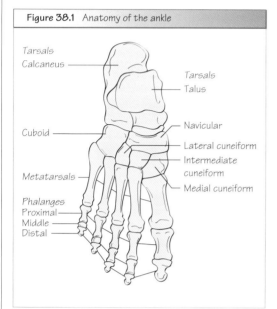

Tarsals
Calcaneus
Tarsals
Talus
Cuboid
Navicular
Lateral cuneiform
Intermediate cuneiform
Metatarsals
Medial cuneiform
Phalanges
Proximal
Middle
Distal

Figure 38.2 Ottawa foot and ankle X-ray guidelines

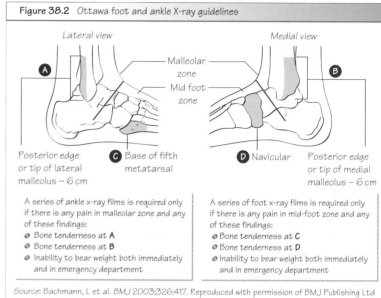

Lateral view
Medial view
Malleolar zone
Mid foot zone
Posterior edge or tip of lateral malleolus – 6 cm
Base of fifth metatarsal
Navicular
Posterior edge or tip of medial malleolus – 6 cm

A series of ankle x-ray films is required only if there is any pain in malleolar zone and any of these findings:
- Bone tenderness at **A**
- Bone tenderness at **B**
- Inability to bear weight both immediately and in emergency department

A series of foot x-ray films is required only if there is any pain in mid-foot zone and any of these findings:
- Bone tenderness at **C**
- Bone tenderness at **D**
- Inability to bear weight both immediately and in emergency department

Source: Bachmann, L et al. BMJ 2003;326:417. Reproduced with permission of BMJ Publishing Ltd

Figure 38.3 Medial/deltoid ligament complex

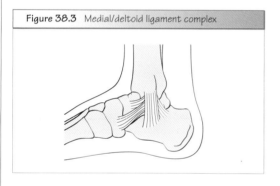

Figure 38.4 Lateral ligament

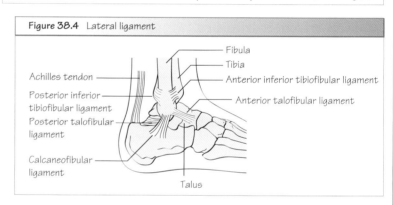

Fibula
Tibia
Achilles tendon
Anterior inferior tibiofibular ligament
Posterior inferior tibiofibular ligament
Anterior talofibular ligament
Posterior talofibular ligament
Calcaneofibular ligament
Talus

Figure 38.5 Weber classification. Weber A below the syndesmosis, Weber B at the syndesmosis, Weber C above the syndesmosis

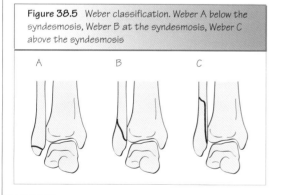

A   B   C

Figure 38.6 Widening of the space between the talus and medial malleolus, known as the 'talar shift', can often be very subtle. Need full-length lower leg views

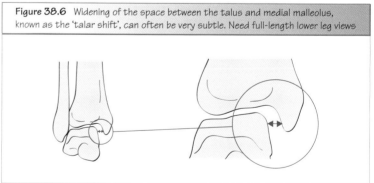

The ankle is made up of the distal tibia and fibula, which along with the talus forms a mortise-type joint. The ankle is secured to the foot by ligaments, which are vital to the joint's stability but are also very commonly injured. The Achilles tendon is also an important structure associated with the ankle and should be included within the assessment.

General approach to the patient

Take a detailed history of the mechanism of injury inversion (foot turning in) or eversion (foot turning out) or hyper dorsiflexion. Was it during sports? If so, what sport? Did it involve a tackle during football or landing from a jump in basketball? Was it a twisting injury with foot staying firmly planted but the body or lower leg twisting, such as in snowboarding? Were they able to walk straight away? Did they continue playing? Was the swelling immediate or slow onset?

Assess whether the patient can walk; take note if they are in a wheelchair, limping or hopping. *Look* at the whole of the lower leg from the knee down, including the foot, removing socks and shoes. Assess for any bruising, swelling, wounds, deformity. Starting at the knee, *feel* down the full length of the fibula and tibia, paying particular attention to the proximal fibula head. Palpate the medial/lateral malleoli and associated ligaments. Check the calcaneum, navicular and base of fifth metatarsal. Ensure you palpate the Achilles tendon and assess for any tenderness or step/gap within the tendon. *Move* – check the range of movement (up and down (dorsiflexion and plantar flexion). Assess the integrity of the Achilles by performing the calf squeeze test (see Chapter 37). Check the dorsal pedis and posterior tibial pulses and sensation of the foot.

When to X-ray

Use the Ottawa ankle/foot rules to assess whether the patient requires an X-ray of the ankle or foot or in some cases both. If the patient cannot weight-bear they need an X-ray. If there is bony tenderness over the posterior aspect of the lateral or medial malleolus, the base of the fifth metacarpal or the navicular, an X-ray is required. Tenderness over the calcaneum after a fall from a height needs an X-ray. This rule does not apply to patients over the age of 55, or to children under the age of 15 (see Figure 38.2). However, the 'rules' are guidelines and the clinician must use their judgement, mechanism of injury and clinical findings. If the patient has attended previously and an X-ray was not deemed necessary but the patient is still having pain and reduced function more than 72 h post-injury, then X-ray.

Injuries
Sprains

The term 'ankle sprain' covers a wide spectrum of soft tissue injuries ranging from minor to major damage of the lateral ligament complex. Most patients have simple sprains, where the tenderness is localised over the anterior slip of the lateral ligament and the patient can walk. These injuries are treated sympathetically with rest, ice, analgesia and elevation. Patients with more significant symptoms and findings who cannot weight-bear may require a range of different interventions (e.g. physiotherapy, immobilisation and further imaging).

Fractures

A deformed dislocated ankle should be relocated immediately without waiting for radiographs to confirm the diagnosis and then immobilised in plaster and X-rays taken. Always assess the neurovascular status of the foot pre and post manipulation and then refer to the orthopaedic team.

Fracture of the ankle can involve either the lateral or medial malleolus or both (bimalleolar fractures). A trimalleolar is one that involves both the lateral and medial malleolus as well as the posterior distal portion of the tibia (the posterior malleolus).

With fractures of the lateral malleolus the Weber classification is often used (see Figure 38.5). Patients with Weber type A fractures, where the fracture is below the ankle mortise, are considered to have stable injuries. Therefore, single closed undisplaced fractures of the malleoli that are considered stable can be treated conservatively in a plaster of Paris with a review in fracture clinic.

Weber type B and C fractures along with patients with bi/trimalleolar fractures should be considered to have unstable injuries and require referral to the orthopaedic team.

Other fractures within the ankle can involve the talus; these can be osteochondral fractures of the talar dome. These result from a compressive force following an inversion/eversion type injury and are common in young to middle-aged adults. On X-ray they appear as an indentation (cortical defect) usually over superior–lateral aspect of the talus on the anterior–posterior mortise view.

A common finding on X-ray interpretation is small avulsion fractures of the anterior aspect of the talus; they are usually due to repetitive minor trauma and are often seen in footballers.

High-energy trauma can sometimes result in fractures to the neck or body of the talus. Although these fractures are rare, owing to its vascular supply they are at greater risk of avascular necrosis, and urgent orthopaedic review should be organised.

 Diagnoses not to be missed

Achilles tendon rupture

Always examine the integrity of this tendon when examining a patient with an ankle injury.

Talar shift

When reviewing X-rays of the ankle, check for the presence of talar shift. The talus fits snugly within the ankle mortise. X-rays should confirm that it is equidistant from the lateral malleolus, the tibia above and the medial malleolus. When shifted, the talus moves laterally away from the medial malleolus leaving a larger than normal gap. Talar shift is commonly seen in patients with unstable bi/trimalleolar fractures. When talar shift is recognised without any obvious fractures, suspect a maisonneuve injury, where there is diastasis (widening) of the inferior tib/fib joint and a high fibula fracture. An X-ray of the whole leg is required. See Figure 38.6.

Fractured calcaneum

A crush fracture of the calcaneum following a fall from a height may give rise to bimalleolar swelling and be mistaken for an ankle injury. Always look at the calcaneum on the lateral X-ray to exclude a fracture.

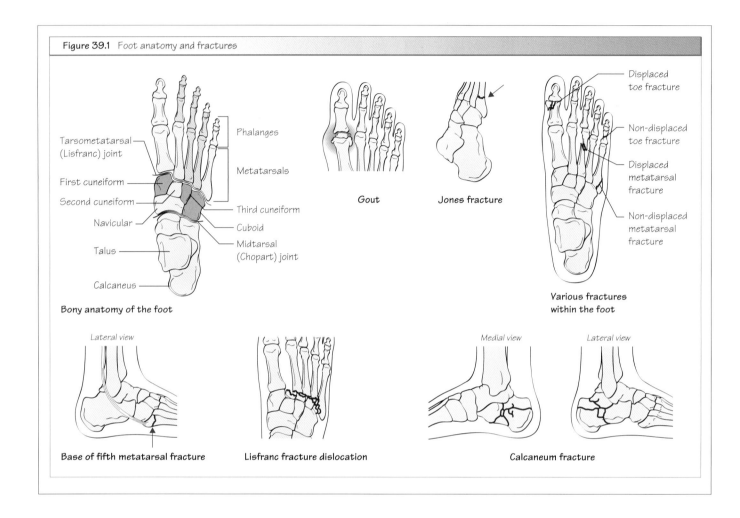

Figure 39.1 Foot anatomy and fractures

Tarsometatarsal (Lisfranc) joint

First cuneiform

Second cuneiform

Navicular

Talus

Calcaneus

Phalanges

Metatarsals

Third cuneiform

Cuboid

Midtarsal (Chopart) joint

Bony anatomy of the foot

Gout

Jones fracture

Displaced toe fracture

Non-displaced toe fracture

Displaced metatarsal fracture

Non-displaced metatarsal fracture

Various fractures within the foot

Lateral view

Base of fifth metatarsal fracture

Lisfranc fracture dislocation

Medial view

Lateral view

Calcaneum fracture

Minor Injury and Minor Illness at a Glance, First Edition. Edited by Francis Morris, Jim Wardrope, and Shammi Ramlakhan.

90 © 2014 John Wiley & Sons, Ltd. Published 2014 by John Wiley & Sons, Ltd. Companion Website: www.ataglanceseries.com/minorinjury

The foot is made up of 26 bones and is divided into the forefoot (metatarsals and phalanges), the mid-foot (navicular, cuboid and cuneiforms) and the hind foot (calcaneum and talus). Its main function is to support the body's weight and is essential for walking and running. Patients frequently present with traumatic and non-traumatic foot problems related to pain and/or loss of function.

Approach to the patient

Elicit the mechanism of injury. Was it a simple 'went over on my foot'? If playing sports, were they able to play on? Was there a history of a fall/jump from a height or history of long distance walking/running? Take note of any medications, as some drugs are associated with gout. *Look* – note the gait and whether the patient is walking/limping/hopping or is in a wheelchair. *Look* for any swelling/bruising/wounds or obvious deformity. Feel the bones of the ankle and Achilles tendon region. Systemically work across the foot to include the calcaneum, talus, navicular, cuboid, cuneiforms, metatarsals and toes. Always check the neurovascular status by assessing the peripheral pulses, capillary refill and the sensation.

If considering X-ray, refer to the Ottawa ankle and foot rules (see Chapter 38); however, remember the rules are guidelines and should not replace clinical judgement. The normal radiographs obtained are a dorsal plantar view and an oblique view. Occasionally you will need to request a true lateral if there is tenderness or severe swelling within the mid foot region, or an axial calcaneal view in suspected calcaneum fractures.

Specific injuries

Fifth metatarsal fracture

A twisting or sudden inversion of the foot results in a sudden pulling and tightening of the peroneus brevis tendon resulting in an avulsion fracture of the base of the fifth metatarsal. These fractures are usually treated symptomatically with a support bandage if the patient is able to weight-bear or a plaster cast backslab if unable to weight-bear. Alternatively, the patient can sustain a 'Jones' fracture, which is a transverse fracture that occurs approximately 1.5–2 cm distal to the tuberosity and requires plaster immobilisation.

Crush injuries

These can occur when either a heavy weight is dropped onto or rolled over the foot. This may result in significant pain and swelling and may include fractures of one or more metatarsal shafts. Great care needs to be taken with crush injuries, particularly if there is severe swelling, pain and generalised tenderness, as compartment syndrome needs to be considered and the patient may need admission for elevation and close observation.

Stress fracture

The metatarsals are the commonest site for a stress fracture, sometimes referred to as a 'march' or 'fatigue' fracture. They result from repeated or continuous stress, such as running or significant walking. The fracture usually occurs in the neck of the second/third metatarsal and appears as a hairline fracture with no displacement. In the early stages the fracture is often not visible. If the patient gives a good history and is symptomatic with localised tenderness over the metatarsal shaft then they should be reviewed in 7–10 days and possibly re-X-rayed to observe for any periosteal reaction or callus formation at the fracture site. Treatment is by simple analgesia and reduction in activity.

Toes

Injuries to the toes are common; when they occur in the second to fifth toes X-ray is not usually indicated as it does not alter management. However, if there is an associated wound over the potential fracture site or severe deformity then X-ray as compound fractures will need prophylactic antibiotics and displaced fractures or dislocations will require manipulation. Injuries to the great toe are more significant; these should always be X-rayed and followed up in fracture clinic.

Calcaneum

Fractures to the calcaneum are usually caused by falling or jumping from a considerable height and landing on the heels. The fractures are often bilateral and the patient should be thoroughly assessed as they can often have associated injuries of the knees or spine. If a calcaneum fracture is suspected then an axial calcaneal view should be requested. Any disruption of the trabecular pattern may indicate a subtle fracture; a sclerotic line may be seen in subtle impacted fractures. Referral to orthopaedics is indicated.

Other bones

Fractures to the navicular and cuboid are often avulsion-type fractures and should be treated symptomatically. Significant fractures require a below-knee backslab and follow-up.

Non-traumatic foot problems

Plantar fasciitis

The patient presents with no history of trauma but complains of pain in the sole of their heel. There is usually no swelling or erythema and it is often worse first thing in the morning or after rest and on weight-bearing. Localised tenderness may be present on palpation of the heel and plantar fascia. Exercises, a heel raise and analgesia are the mainstays of treatment.

Gout

Sudden onset of severe pain, redness and swelling in the first metatarsalphalangeal joint with no history of trauma is suggestive of acute gout. The patient may have had previous attacks or give a history of heavy alcohol intake or diuretic therapy. If gout is suspected, treat with nonsteroidal anti-inflammatory drugs and refer the patient to their GP.

Metatarsalgia

This is the name given to pain arising from the heads of your metatarsal bones. It can be associated with a number of different conditions affecting the foot. Common causes include overuse, wearing high heels, being overweight and 'Morton's neuroma'.

> ▶ **Diagnoses not to be missed**
>
> **Lisfranc injury**
>
> The 'tarsometatarsal dislocation' results from either forced dorsiflexion of the foot or forced inversion/eversion of the forefoot with the hind foot fixed. Clinically, the patient's foot will be very swollen and bruised and they will be unable to weight-bear. Radiographically, the clinician needs to assess alignment of the base of the metatarsals and cuneiforms.
>
> **Ischaemia**
>
> Always assess the foot pulses in a patient with foot pain and look for evidence of vascular insufficiency.

40 Approach to the injured child

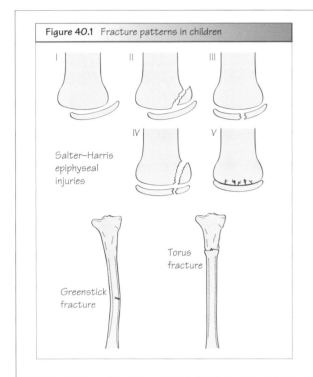

Figure 40.1 Fracture patterns in children

Salter–Harris epiphyseal injuries (I, II, III, IV, V)

Greenstick fracture

Torus fracture

Table 40.1 Presentations where non-accidental injury should be considered

History	• Inadequate supervision • Unexplained injury • Delayed presentation • Injury inconsistent with stated mechanism • Injury developmentally incompatible • Explanation changes • Frequent attendances for minor/vague reasons • If family is known to be at risk
Examination	• Parents/carer unconcerned or aggressive • Evidence of older injuries which are unexplained • Bruises away from bony prominences (cheek, base of neck, back, buttocks, trunk and arms) • Imprint of implement or hand • Large bruises or clusters • Perineal injury • Burns in glove/stocking distribution • Circular (cigarette) burns • Fractures in pre-mobile children (under 18 months) • Humeral/femoral fractures in under 3 year old

Minor Injury and Minor Illness at a Glance, First Edition. Edited by Francis Morris, Jim Wardrope, and Shammi Ramlakhan.

92 © 2014 John Wiley & Sons, Ltd. Published 2014 by John Wiley & Sons, Ltd. Companion Website: www.ataglanceseries.com/minorinjury

General approach

Children differ from adults not only in how they manifest injury or illness, but also in their ability to communicate symptoms or even the site of an injury. Their developmental stage may also pose diagnostic and management challenges; for example, assessment of a child before they can talk depends entirely on parental history and examination. They may have stranger anxiety or an illogical (to an adult!) misconception of a clinician's intentions or of their illness. Adolescents may be widely variable on how they respond to injury or illness – some may be mature/logical while others may have exaggerated and even hysterical responses to relatively minor injury/illness.

A non-threatening approach is obviously important. With younger children, maintain some distance initially until they can be assured that the clinician poses no threat. It is best to maintain eye contact at their level and speak to them using age-appropriate language.

Early and adequate analgesia is very important as often this can result in a dramatic improvement in symptoms and facilitates a more meaningful assessment.

Examination

Particularly with younger children, physical contact should be avoided until they are comfortable with your presence or for as long as possible. Much information can be gained by simple observation; for example, children with pulled elbows (Chapter 29) tend to hold their arms in a particular position. Similarly, swelling, erythema, bruising, asymmetry, range of movement or a limp can all be elicited by observation. Exposure is important and it is often better to ask parents/carers to undress the child when the clinician is not in the room or while the history is being elicited.

It is often useful to allow toddlers and younger children to remain seated on parents/carers while being examined. The use of distractions/toys helps with minimising their anxiety and makes examination easier. Letting them handle instruments may also assist in reducing anxiety.

Examining the unaffected limb or a site distant from the area of concern first may help put the child at ease. Often, it is necessary to examine an entire limb if the site of injury is uncertain; for example, starting at the clavicle if a wrist injury is suspected and vice versa.

It is not uncommon for the site of an injury to still be uncertain even after physical examination. Unnecessary or whole-limb radiological investigation should be avoided, and it is sometimes best to reassess the child after a period of observation and analgesia as this can make the diagnosis more clear.

Injury patterns

There are several characteristic injury patterns in children that are related to their skeletal development, and which are not seen in adults.

Epiphyseal injury

Epiphyseal injuries account for up to 15% of paediatric long bone fractures. They range from subtle slips (see Salter–Harris classification) (Figure 40.1) to impacted injuries which can result in significant deformity in later life. Recognition of these injuries is important as they can be easily missed if the clinician is unaware of the patterns.

Greenstick fractures

A child's bone is softer and more pliable than adults. In addition, the periosteum is thicker and more restrictive. This means that bones may bend and only partially break, analogous to a greenstick. Often the periosteum remains intact on one side of the fracture (Figure 40.1). Occasionally, the bone bends and causes bowing without a fracture being visible.

Buckle/torus fractures

These are a type of greenstick fracture where the soft bone is compressed, and causes buckling of the cortex/periosteum (Figure 40.1). These are common around the wrist, and most children do well with conservative treatment.

Toddlers' fractures

These are often innocuous injuries to the tibia which present with refusal to weight-bear after a fall or relatively minor trauma. There may be tenderness to the mid-distal tibia or pain on axial compression. The fracture is usually an undisplaced spiral injury, but initial X-rays are usually normal in appearance. Treatment with an above-knee plaster for at least 10 days is routine, at which point repeat X-ray may demonstrate periosteal reaction confirming the fracture.

Non-accidental injury

Clinicians should be alert to the possibility of an injury in any child being non-accidental. Clues in the history include delayed presentation, changing explanation or inconsistent history, developmentally implausible mechanism (e.g. neonate rolling off a bed) or denial of injury.

Unexplained bruising in unusual areas (mouth, base of neck, back, genitalia) or of varying ages should prompt further evaluation for abuse. Similarly, patterns of bruising (from hand/fingers or other objects) or burns (cigarette, glove/stocking distribution) are significant.

Any injury in a non-mobile infant which is either unexplained or has an inadequate accidental explanation is cause for concern.

If a clinician has any concerns regarding non-accidental injury in a child, they are mandated to act on that concern in line with local child protection policies.

Prescribing for children

Children, and in particular neonates, differ from adults in how they respond and metabolise drugs; therefore, particular care should be taken when prescribing medication. Most drugs doses are calculated on a weight basis, and the correct dose and frequency should be confirmed with a formulary if the clinician is unfamiliar or unsure.

41 The limping child

Common causes of the limping child classed by age
Toddler age 0–3 years
● Septic joint
● Osteomyelitis
● Developmental hip dysplasia
● Toddler's fracture
● Transient synovitis
Child 3–10 years
● Transient synovitis
● Septic joint
● Osteomyelitis
● Perthes' disease
● Juvenile rheumatoid arthritis
Older child >10 years
● Slipped upper femoral epiphysis
● Septic joint
● Osteomyelitis
● Soft tissue injury
Other less common causes presenting at any age
● Non-accidental injury must always be considered.
● Malignancies: leukaemia, lymphoma, Ewing's sarcoma
● Neuromuscular disorders: muscular dystrophy, cerebral palsy, peripheral neuropathies

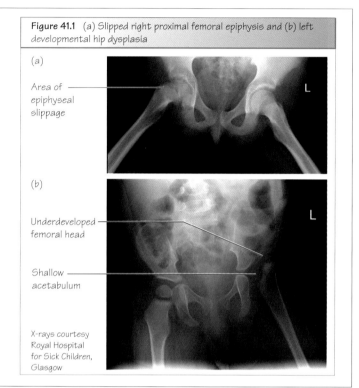

Figure 41.1 (a) Slipped right proximal femoral epiphysis and (b) left developmental hip dysplasia

(a)

Area of epiphyseal slippage

(b)

Underdeveloped femoral head

Shallow acetabulum

X-rays courtesy Royal Hospital for Sick Children, Glasgow

Approach to the child

When assessing a child with a limp there is a wide range of differential diagnoses to consider. Most of these are benign and self-limiting; however, a few can be serious and even life threatening. A limp is defined as an abnormal gait pattern secondary to pain, weakness or deformity. A detailed history should be obtained through consultation with parents or carers. It is important to remember that a child's walking pattern is not fully developed until the age of 7 years and so a history must detect a change in gait as the key feature of concern. The history should focus on the following:

- onset of limp and frequency/recurrence of symptoms;
- recent trauma;
- birth and developmental history;
- systemic enquiry (recent acute illness).

Even an innocuous fall in a child can cause a limp. Children have supple joints with developing bones and growth plates which are prone to sprains, subluxation, fractures and even dislocation. Examination of the child involves:

- **Look.** Observe the stance and gait pattern for the degree of limp. The child should be fully undressed and carefully examined to reveal any obvious trauma (bruises, swelling and deformity). A simple foreign body in the sole of the foot can be an easily treated cause of a limp, but it often gets missed if a thorough examination is not carried out. Erythema particularly over a joint should be noted.
- **Feel.** Palpate the joints and limbs for any bony tenderness or swelling. Each joint should be examined in turn. Assess the skin temperature and ease with which the joints can passively be moved. Note how comfortable the child is throughout. Children can be a challenge to examine, and so distraction techniques may help.
- **Move.** The hips should be moved symmetrically looking at internal rotation in particular as it is a sensitive marker of hip joint pathology. Joints should be actively and passively moved and the range noted.

Further examination of the abdomen, groin, spine and genital area should be performed.

Box 41.1 lists the common causes of a limp in children according to age.

Minor Injury and Minor Illness at a Glance, First Edition. Edited by Francis Morris, Jim Wardrope, and Shammi Ramlakhan.

94 © 2014 John Wiley & Sons, Ltd. Published 2014 by John Wiley & Sons, Ltd. Companion Website: www.ataglanceseries.com/minorinjury

Specific conditions

Septic arthritis

This is a serious condition resulting from infection within the joint space. Common pathogens include *Staphylococcus aureus*. It usually occurs as a result of haematogenous bacterial spread. This condition must be excluded in any child presenting with a limp. If left untreated, growth arrest and joint destruction can occur. It is not always easy to detect and exclude; however, children with a septic joint usually (though not always) appear toxic. The presence of fever, joint pain, elevated erythrocyte sedimentation rate, C-reactive protein and elevated white cell count is suggestive. These five parameters can be used to predict the presence of a septic joint, with three or more giving an 80% chance of joint infection. Definitive investigation would involve ultrasound and joint aspiration. The child would require intravenous antibiotics and urgent referral to an orthopaedic surgeon for surgical wash out of the joint.

Irritable hip/transient synovitis

This presents between the ages of 3 and 10 years and is the most common cause of atraumatic hip pain. The history is often (but not always) of a mild viral illness in the preceding weeks. Diagnosis is confirmed by ultrasound of the hip revealing a joint effusion, although this is not always necessary. Other more serious conditions must be excluded before this diagnosis is made. A child with a transient synovitis is not toxic and can usually weight-bear. Symptoms will resolve within 2 weeks. The child should be prescribed a course of nonsteroidal anti-inflammatory medication and followed up until complete resolution of symptoms. If this diagnosis is made, the parents must be warned of red flag symptoms and advised to re-present if concern arises.

Perthes' disease

This typically occurs in boys aged 4–8 years and is a result of avascular necrosis of the femoral head. The child may have a long history of intermittent limp that becomes more persistent. Plain X-ray can confirm the diagnosis; however, technetium bone scan or magnetic resonance imaging may be required. Treatment is by surgical or non-surgical means under the care of an orthopaedic specialist.

Slipped upper femoral epiphysis

This mostly presents in children over 10 years of age; however, it should be considered in younger children, especially in overweight boys. X-ray findings are of a displaced proximal femoral epiphysis in relation to the metaphysis (Figure 41.1). Referred pain is commonly felt in the knee joint, and the diagnosis should be considered in children presenting with knee pain without abnormal findings. If the slip is subtle then it can be missed on plain X-rays, and so a frog's leg lateral view should be obtained. Orthopaedic referral is required.

Toddler's fracture

This injury is commonly seen after an innocuous fall in pre-school children. The diagnosis should be suspected in a child who has localised tenderness over the distal tibia. Initial X-rays may be normal; however, the child usually has a limp and history of mild trauma. In the context of negative X-rays and after exclusion of other causes of a limp, the child should be immobilised in plaster and reviewed again in 10 days' time. At this stage, periosteal reaction is usually evident on X-ray.

 Diagnoses not to be missed

Unexplained musculoskeletal symptoms and recurrent presentations must be taken seriously.

In any presentation of a limping child, if no conclusion is made at the time of initial presentation then it is imperative that appropriate follow-up is arranged.

Malignancy

A careful, methodical approach is vital in order to detect the possibility of underlying malignancy. The presence of non-articular bone pain, night sweats, weight loss, fever, fatigue and pallor are all suggestive of malignancy and investigations should be tailored accordingly.

Non-accidental injury

This may present with a limp. Children should be undressed to be fully examined. Possible features of non-accidental injury include delay in presentation, mismatch in history between carer and child, bruises of varying ages and certain patterns of bruises. Alarms should be raised to initiate further assessment.

Non-articular causes

As well as the musculoskeletal causes of a limp, it is essential to remember that other common paediatric conditions can present with a limp (e.g. acute appendicitis, testicular torsion).

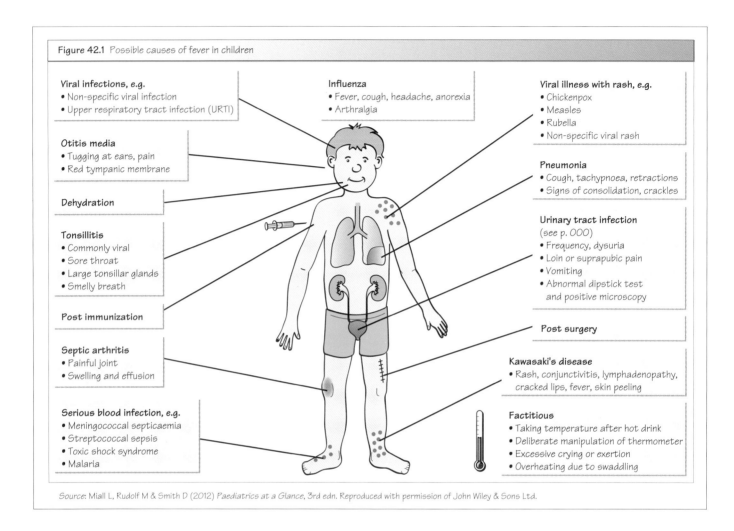

Figure 42.1 Possible causes of fever in children

Viral infections, e.g.
- Non-specific viral infection
- Upper respiratory tract infection (URTI)

Otitis media
- Tugging at ears, pain
- Red tympanic membrane

Dehydration

Tonsillitis
- Commonly viral
- Sore throat
- Large tonsillar glands
- Smelly breath

Post immunization

Septic arthritis
- Painful joint
- Swelling and effusion

Serious blood infection, e.g.
- Meningococcal septicaemia
- Streptococcal sepsis
- Toxic shock syndrome
- Malaria

Influenza
- Fever, cough, headache, anorexia
- Arthralgia

Viral illness with rash, e.g.
- Chickenpox
- Measles
- Rubella
- Non-specific viral rash

Pneumonia
- Cough, tachypnoea, retractions
- Signs of consolidation, crackles

Urinary tract infection
(see p. 000)
- Frequency, dysuria
- Loin or suprapubic pain
- Vomiting
- Abnormal dipstick test and positive microscopy

Post surgery

Kawasaki's disease
- Rash, conjunctivitis, lymphadenopathy, cracked lips, fever, skin peeling

Factitious
- Taking temperature after hot drink
- Deliberate manipulation of thermometer
- Excessive crying or exertion
- Overheating due to swaddling

Source: Miall L, Rudolf M & Smith D (2012) Paediatrics at a Glance, 3rd edn. Reproduced with permission of John Wiley & Sons Ltd.

Minor Injury and Minor Illness at a Glance, First Edition. Edited by Francis Morris, Jim Wardrope, and Shammi Ramlakhan.

General approach

Fever is one of the most common paediatric presentations to unplanned care. The majority of children will not have a serious cause for their illness; however, there are many significant causes of fever that should not be missed. The variation in signs and symptoms across the paediatric population means that detecting more dangerous infections can be quite tricky. The aim should be to find a focus for the fever and to exclude possible serious explanations for the child's symptoms. If this cannot be done then seek a more senior opinion or refer the child for paediatric assessment.

A thorough history from the parents (and the child if appropriate) can give many clues. Reported fever at home (whether measured or not) should be taken as significant, even if the child is afebrile on examination. Take note of nonspecific symptoms and do not dismiss the parent's assessment of their child ('he's really not right').

A full set of observations should be recorded and the child should be undressed fully so that you can examine every system and be certain that you have not missed any petechial spots, peeling skin or joint abnormalities. In the majority of children the cause of fever is a self-limiting viral illness (upper respiratory tract infection, flu-like illness, gastroenteritis) that will resolve with supportive care from the parents; this can usually be determined from a thorough history and examination. Figure 42.1 outlines causes of fever that should be considered.

If there is a clear focus for the infection and the child is well then you may consider discharging them home with appropriate advice.

If the child is clearly unwell then you must provide resuscitative treatment and involve specialist teams early. Administration of empirical antibiotics (depending on the suspected source of infection) should ideally happen after culture samples have been taken, but do not delay giving antibiotics in severe illness.

History

This should focus on the duration and nature of illness. In addition, a reported history of fever is significant, even if the temperature is normal when assessed.

A review of symptoms relating to all systems may give clues as to the source of fever. Feeding, hydration and behaviour should be noted to assess severity of the illness. Any recent antibiotics or use of antipyretics should be determined as these may alter the presentation in some cases.

A birth history, any medical conditions (identify high-risk groups) and vaccination history should be taken. Any contacts with ill persons or recent travel should be established.

Examination

Completely undress the child for a full systemic examination. On general examination it should be apparent if they look well or unwell, and whether are they playing and interacting normally. Consider whether they appear subdued, drowsy or irritable, and if the child handles well.

A full set of physiological observations (heart rate, respiratory rate, oxygen saturation, temperature, capillary refill time) should be recorded.

The airway should be examined for stridor or drooling, which may point to potential compromise.

Respiratory examination is undertaken to look for signs of distress, wheeze and crepitations. During the cardiovascular examination it is important to note perfusion quality and hydration status, such as cool extremities, dry lips and tongue, sunken eyes and reduced skin turgor. Listening for murmurs, which may indicate endocarditis is also important. A flow murmur is common in children with fever, however, and if this is found then follow-up after the acute illness to check for resolution is warranted.

Check for abdominal tenderness and organomegaly, and include a check of the external genitalia.

Neurological examination, looking in particular for irritability, meningism, photophobia, bulging fontanelles and changed behaviour.

Ear, nose and throat examination is important as the majority of children will have an upper respiratory tract infection; therefore, you must get a look at pharynx/tonsils and ear drums.

The skin is fully examined for petechial rashes, other rashes, skin infections and jaundice.

Check the limbs, joint and spine for pain on moving/palpation, any abnormal gait, swelling or heat.

Lymphadenopathy is common in young children, and should be examined for, as persistent fever with lymphadenopathy may point to other conditions, such as Kawasaki disease or neoplasia.

Safe discharge

If you have identified the cause of the fever, the child looks well and you have not identified any 'amber' or 'red' flags then you can be reassured. As part of a safe discharge consider the social and family circumstances and the level of parental anxiety and experience. Share your diagnosis with parents and give them information about appropriate use of antipyretics and any other treatment you are providing. Giving clear advice to parents about when to seek medical help (ideally written as well as verbal) is crucial for a safe discharge.

⚑ Diagnoses not to be missed

Febrile child under 5 without a focus

The traffic light system to aid the identification of serious infection in children under 5 without a focus was developed by NICE and is used in the UK (see Figure 42.2). If a child has any 'amber' or 'red' features they should be referred to paediatrics for observation and investigation.

Young infants

Beware of non-specific symptoms such as poor feeding or unsettled behaviour in the young infant – they may be due to serious bacterial infection. Children do not start fully producing their own antibodies until about 6 months of age and so are vulnerable to severe bacterial infections during this period, especially in the first 12 weeks of life. They may not present with typical features of infection in the history or on examination, and it is important to seek a senior opinion or paediatric review for all young infants with nonspecific symptoms. Please note that neonates with sepsis may have hypothermia rather than a fever.

Figure 42.2 Traffic light system for identiying risk of serious illness*

	Green – low risk	Amber – intermediate risk	Red – high risk
Colour (of skin, lips or tongue)	Normal colour	Pallor reported by parent/carer	Pale/mottled/ashen/blue
Activity	Responds normally to social cues Content/smiles Stays awake or awakens quickly Strong normal cry/not crying	Not responding normally to social cues No smile Wakes only with prolonged stimulation Decreased activity	No response to social cues Appears ill to a healthcare professional Does not wake or if roused does not stay awake Weak, high-pitched or continuous cry
Respiratory		Nasal flaring Tachypnoea: – RR > 50 breaths/minute, age 6–12 months – RR > 40 breaths/minute, age > 12 months Oxygen saturation ≤ 95% in air Crackles in the chest	Grunting Tachypnoea: – RR > 60 breaths/minute Moderate or severe chest indrawing
Circulation and hydration	Normal skin and eyes Moist mucous membranes	Tachycardia: – > 160 beats/minute, age < 12 months – > 150 beats/minute, age 12–24 months – > 140 beats/minute, age 2–5 years CRT ≥ 3 seconds Dry mucous membranes Poor feeding in infants Reduced urine output	Reduced skin turgor
Other	None of the amber or red symptoms or signs	Age 3–6 months, temperature ≥ 39°C Fever for ≥ 5 days Rigors Swelling of a limb or joint Non-weight bearing limb/not using an extremity	Age < 3 months, temperature ≥ 38°C Non-blanching rash Bulging fontanelle Neck stiffness Status epilepticus Focal neurological signs Focal seizures

CRT, capillary refill time; RR, respiratory rate

* This traffic light table should be used in conjunction with the recommendations in the guideline on investigations and initial management in children with fever. See http://guidance.nice.org.uk/CG160 (update of NICE clinical guideline 47)

National Institute for Health and Clinical Excellence (2013) CG 160 Feverish illness in children: assessment and initial management of children younger than 5 years. London: NICE. Available from http://guidance.nice.org.uk/CG160 Reproduced with permission.

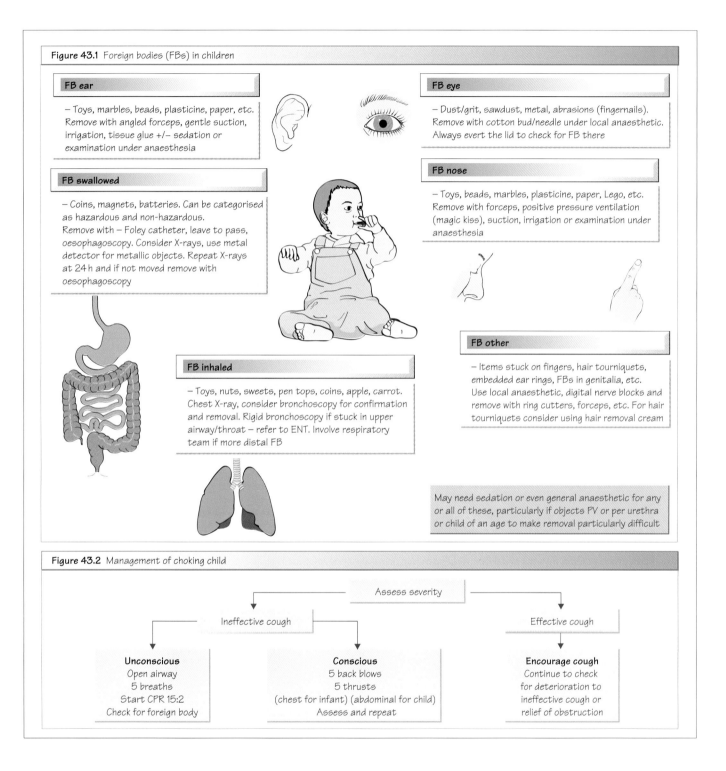

Figure 43.1 Foreign bodies (FBs) in children

FB ear

– Toys, marbles, beads, plasticine, paper, etc. Remove with angled forceps, gentle suction, irrigation, tissue glue +/– sedation or examination under anaesthesia

FB swallowed

– Coins, magnets, batteries. Can be categorised as hazardous and non-hazardous.
Remove with – Foley catheter, leave to pass, oesophagoscopy. Consider X-rays, use metal detector for metallic objects. Repeat X-rays at 24 h and if not moved remove with oesophagoscopy

FB inhaled

– Toys, nuts, sweets, pen tops, coins, apple, carrot. Chest X-ray, consider bronchoscopy for confirmation and removal. Rigid bronchoscopy if stuck in upper airway/throat – refer to ENT. Involve respiratory team if more distal FB

FB eye

– Dust/grit, sawdust, metal, abrasions (fingernails). Remove with cotton bud/needle under local anaesthetic. Always evert the lid to check for FB there

FB nose

– Toys, beads, marbles, plasticine, paper, Lego, etc. Remove with forceps, positive pressure ventilation (magic kiss), suction, irrigation or examination under anaesthesia

FB other

– Items stuck on fingers, hair tourniquets, embedded ear rings, FBs in genitalia, etc.
Use local anaesthetic, digital nerve blocks and remove with ring cutters, forceps, etc. For hair tourniquets consider using hair removal cream

May need sedation or even general anaesthetic for any or all of these, particularly if objects PV or per urethra or child of an age to make removal particularly difficult

Figure 43.2 Management of choking child

Assess severity

Ineffective cough — Effective cough

Unconscious
Open airway
5 breaths
Start CPR 15:2
Check for foreign body

Conscious
5 back blows
5 thrusts
(chest for infant) (abdominal for child)
Assess and repeat

Encourage cough
Continue to check
for deterioration to
ineffective cough or
relief of obstruction

Approach to the child

Children tend to explore the world with their mouths and fingers, and foreign bodies (FBs) are often experimentally placed where they should not. Under the age of 3–4 years this is a particular problem.

Especially for FBs in ears, nose, oropharynx, one gentle attempt at removal should be made generally by non-specialists. Another attempt (senior) may be allowed; then consider the need for sedation or referral/general anaesthetic.

Once removed, always check that the FB has gone, and also that no damage/bleeding has been caused. Always check up the opposite nostril or in the opposite ear!

Successful FB removal requires:
• Reassurance/anxiolysis – talk to the child and parents first and gain their confidence.
• Good positioning, lighting and a helpful assistant are critical.
• The right tools for each job (e.g. speculum for the nose/ear). Jobson–Horn probes, angled forceps, suction, tissue glue, Foley catheters, cotton buds and splinter forceps make a difference.

Success depends on the site and nature of the FB. For example, deep in the external auditory meatus is difficult. Paper disintegrates and is difficult to remove easily in one go. Smooth round beads are difficult to grasp with forceps and may require suction or a hook placed behind the FB to move it forwards.

Specific conditions
Ingested foreign bodies

Most FBs require an anterior–posterior chest X-ray (CXR) and consideration of abdominal X-ray (AXR)/soft tissue lateral neck. If an ingested FB is clearly stuck in the upper oesophagus and is non-hazardous (e.g. a coin), an attempt at removal can be made with a Foley catheter. If this fails, consult a paediatric surgeon.

Hazardous

This includes sharp objects, very large objects, button batteries, more than one magnet. Button batteries are dangerous as the contents are toxic. There is also a danger of local erosion of the mucosa by current passing from the battery, if it is a fresh one. All children who have swallowed a battery should have a CXR (and abdomen if not visible on CXR) to locate the battery as soon as possible. If the battery is in the oesophagus, urgent referral to the paediatric surgeons is needed.

If below the diaphragm, the child can eat and drink normally and the AXR repeated after 12 h. If there is no progress, refer to the surgeons urgently. The battery may have become adherent to the gastric mucosa, leading to a high risk of erosion. If the battery has moved position below the diaphragm and is not fragmenting then the patient can be safely discharged. If the AXR shows that a battery has fragmented or leaked, the patient should be referred immediately to the surgeons for urgent removal. With magnets, the problem is potential adherence across loops of bowel leading to pressure necrosis of bowel wall and perforation.

Non-hazardous

This includes coins, marbles, beads – round, hard, smooth objects. If shown in stomach, allow the child to eat/drink, and repeat X-ray in 12 h. If still in the stomach, then referral to surgeons is warranted.

Do not discharge a child who is coughing, choking or refusing to eat/drink after a suspected ingestion. If there is evidence of complications, X-rays should be requested. A metal detector will pick up aluminium (e.g. can ring-pulls), which may not be seen on an X-ray.

Non-metallic and non-hazardous ingestions can be discharged once eating and drinking OK. Do not instruct parents to 'look for FB in the stools'.

Metallic and non-hazardous – use a metal detector (avoid X-rays). If negative or below the xiphisternum, then can be discharged. If above xiphisternum or equivocal, then an anterior–posterior CXR and AXR/soft tissue lateral neck should be considered.

Foreign body in the nose

If these are visible and easy to remove, then do so. otherwise if unable to remove it, do not have repeat attempts and refer to ear, nose and throat (ENT). Most objects do not require urgent referral the same day. Batteries need urgent removal. A unilateral offensive nasal discharge is strongly suggestive of a long-standing foreign body.

A parental 'magic kiss', irrigation (though most children do not tolerate this well), fine-bore suction, direct removal with forceps or a Jobson–Horne probe are the techniques used. Hard, round objects such as beads can be difficult to get hold and suction.or a hook may be used. Tissue glue on the end of a cotton bud stem can work to fix to a difficult object, removing it once 'set'; however, you need a very still and cooperative patient for this to work.

Foreign body in the ear

Always examine the 'normal' ear first to exclude two FBs and to gain the child's confidence. Remove the FB only if you can do so easily. If it is deep in the ear the chances of success will be low, so have a low threshold for referring. The first attempt will probably be your best chance of success. If attempts fail and the FB is a battery, refer to the ENT team on-call. Otherwise refer to **next ENT clinic** for removal there. Do not make repeated attempts at removal as this distresses the child and makes the ENT job more difficult. For removal, suction (the noise tends to distress small children), a probe, forceps, irrigation or tissue glue (care as above) can be used. Once removed, check that there is no FB remaining and that the tympanic membrane is intact and that there is no trauma/bleeding.

Inhaled foreign body in the airway
Upper airway
• *Complete obstruction.* If there is a complete upper airway obstruction, then manage as per the choking child (Figure 43.2).
• *Partial obstruction.* Needs referral to ENT registrar on-call urgently. Witnessed inhalation or good history of inhalation but no clinical evidence of deterioration of respiratory function still needs urgent referral.
• *Always request CXR* with inhaled FB (looking for collapse), and lateral neck for soft tissues if FB is suspected to be in the neck, irrespective of whether FB is radio-opaque or not.
• Do not turn the partial obstruction into a complete one by distressing the child, forcing them to lie down or attempting inappropriate removal manoeuvres. Nurse them wherever they are most comfortable (often mum's lap) and give oxygen if needed.
• Manage airway, breathing and circulation and get early senior help.

Lower airway
The possibility of an inhaled FB should be borne in mind in young children (age 6 months–4 years are most at risk) who present having had an episode of choking/cyanosis/stridor, altered consciousness, a persistent cough or wheeze, dyspnoea, fever.

Remember, many episodes are unwitnessed – the history may be vague. Sudden onset of symptoms in an otherwise well child with/without a choking episode is usually key.

Differential diagnosis includes all causes of wheeze, cough and respiratory compromise. Consider asthma, bronchiolitis, wheeze-associated viral illness, pneumonias. An FB impacting in the lower airways produces a variety of symptoms and signs but examination may be entirely normal, especially early on.

Management Give **oxygen** if hypoxic; ensure the ABCs are OK; if in any doubt call for senior help. Arrange a CXR (plus lateral X-ray of the neck to show the upper airway if signs or symptoms suggestive). Look for an opaque foreign body, segmental or lobar collapse, localised emphysema/hyper-expansion (due to a ball-valve obstruction effect). The CXR may be completely normal. If in any doubt at all, **refer**.

Foreign body in the eye

See Chapter 14.

▶ Diagnoses not to be missed

Ingested button batteries/magnets

These are potentially dangerous and should be removed acutely or early unless they are clearly transiting the bowel. Beware the instance where a magnet (on its own non-hazardous) is ingested with others. These adhere across adjacent loops of bowel (often small bowel) and perforate.

Foreign body in the eye but none seen

Do not miss the FB under the upper lid, or the alternative FB sensation caused by a dendritic ulcer of herpes simplex virus infection (see Chapter 14).

Non-accidental injury

It is most unusual for children to insert FBs into orifices other than mouth, ears and noses. If there are FBs per vagina/per rectum, consider non-accidental injury or fabricated or factitious illness.

Figure 44.1 Common sites for childhood rashes and lesion morphology

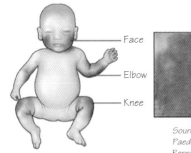

Face

Elbow

Knee

Source: Miall L, Rudolf M & Smith D (2012)
Paediatrics at a Glance, 3rd edn.
Reproduced with permission of John Wiley & Sons Ltd.

Recognizing common skin lesions

Macule
A small (usually less than 1 cm in diameter), flat blemish or discolouration that can be brown, tan, red, or white and has same texture as surrounding skin

Wheal
A slightly raised, firm lesion of variable size and shape, surrounded by edema; skin may be red or pale

Bulla
A raised, thin-walled blister greater than 0.5 cm in diameter, containing clear or serous fluid

Nodule
A small, firm, circumscribed, elevated lesion 1 to 2 cm in diameter with possible skin discolouration

Vesicle
A small (less than 0.5 cm in diameter), thin-walled, raised blister containing clear, serous, purulent, or bloody fluid

Papule
A small, solid, raised lesion less than 1 cm in diameter), with red to purple skin discoloration

Pustule
A circumscribed, pus- or lymph-filled, elevated lesion that varies in diameter and may be firm or soft and white or yellow

Tumor
A solid, raised mass usually larger than 2 cm in diameter with possible skin discoloration

Figure 44.2 Fifth disease

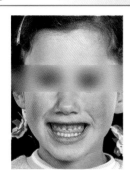

Source: Miall L, Rudolf M & Smith D (2012)
Paediatrics at a Glance, 3rd edn.
Reproduced with permission of John Wiley & Sons Ltd.

Figure 44.5 Erythroderma

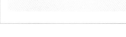

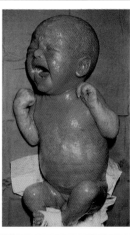

Source: Burns T, Breathnach S, Cox N & Griffiths C (2010)
Rook's Textbook of Dermatology, 8e.
Reproduced with permission of John Wiley & Sons Ltd.

Figure 44.3 Impetigo

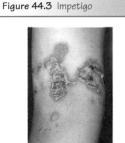

Source: Miall L, Rudolf M & Smith D (2012)
Paediatrics at a Glance, 3rd edn.
Reproduced with permission
of John Wiley & Sons Ltd.

Figure 44.4 Molluscum contagiosum

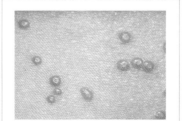

Source: Miall L, Rudolf M & Smith D (2012)
Paediatrics at a Glance, 3rd edn.
Reproduced with permission
of John Wiley & Sons Ltd.

Figure 44.6 Stevens–Johnson

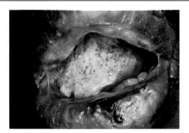

Source: Burns T, Breathnach S, Cox N & Griffiths C (2010)
Rook's Textbook of Dermatology, 8e.
Reproduced with permission of John Wiley & Sons Ltd.

Figure 44.7 Meningococcal septicaemia

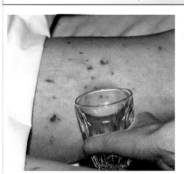

The glass test: Press the side of a clear glass firmly against the skin. A positive test is when the rash does not fade under pressure

Source: Miall L, Rudolf M & Smith D (2012)
Paediatrics at a Glance, 3rd edn.
Reproduced with permission of John Wiley & Sons Ltd.

Minor Injury and Minor Illness at a Glance, First Edition. Edited by Francis Morris, Jim Wardrope, and Shammi Ramlakhan.

Approach to the child

Rashes in children are common and having a structured and pragmatic approach is helpful. The site and duration of the rash, itch, blisters, pain and exacerbating factors are all important.

Past medical and drug history, immunisation history and family history can provide clues to the current problem.

When examining, look at the distribution to determine whether the rash is localised, generalised or symmetrical. Morphology is important with regard to the primary lesion, shape, size, whether raised or flat, margins, surface characteristics and colour (Figure 44.1). It is important to examine as much skin as possible. Look in the mouth and remember to check the hair and the nails.

Specific conditions

Viral exanthems

Exanthem is the term given to a widespread rash that is usually accompanied by systemic symptoms such as fever, headache and malaise. Viral exanthems are mostly associated with self-limited diseases which usually resolve within 10 days.

The most common childhood viral exanthems include measles or rubeola, rubella, varicella (chickenpox), fifth disease and roseola.

Chickenpox (varicella)

This is most common in children under age 10. The first symptom is usually fever, followed in 1–2 days by a rash that can be very itchy. The rash starts with red spots that soon turn into fluid-filled blisters. Some children have only a few blisters while in others it can be florid. These dry and form scabs in 3–5 days' time.

The virus is spread either airborne or by direct person-to-person contact. It develops within 10–21 days of contact with an infected person. It is most contagious on the day before the rash appears.

Complications such as skin infection, pneumonia or central nervous system infection should be borne in mind when assessing a child with chickenpox. Contact with pregnant women or the immunocompromised should be avoided.

Slapped cheek syndrome (fifth disease or erythema infectiosum)

This often starts with a low-grade fever, headache and mild flu-like symptoms with the rash appearing after a few days. Besides red cheeks (which gives this condition its name), a red, lacy rash may also be seen in the upper arms and legs (Figure 44.2). It is caused by parvovirus B19 and is spread via mucus, saliva or blood. It is most common between the ages of 5 and 15. The rash usually lasts 2 days and rarely up to a few weeks. Symptomatic treatment is all that is required; however, the child should avoid pregnant women.

Impetigo

This infection is most common around the nose and mouth, hands and forearms. It is caused by *Staphylococcus aureus*, *Streptococcus pyogenes* or both.

Bullous (large blisters) and non-bullous impetigo (crusted) are the two types, with the latter being more common (Figure 44.3). It is often spread when infected areas of skin are touched and then touching other parts of the body or other persons.

Treatment is with antibiotics, which can be topical if a small area is affected or systemic if the area is large or the child unwell.

Atopic eczema

This is the most common type of eczema, with pruritus the hallmark symptom. The distribution depends on the age of the child (e.g. infants have mainly facial involvement, while older children have flexural).

Treatment involves eliminating precipitating factors (e.g. soaps, irritating clothing and excessive sweating). Emollients are the mainstay of treatment, while topical corticosteroids reduce pruritus and inflammation. Antihistamines are used to minimise itching, while oral antibiotics may be given in short courses to reduce staphylococcal infections. Referral to a dermatologist is recommended in severe cases or if uncontrolled by standard measures.

Molluscum contagiosum

Molluscum contagiosum is a self-limiting viral skin infection. It is transmitted by direct skin-to-skin contact either by auto-inoculation or person-to-person contact and has an incubation period of 1–6 weeks. It is highly contagious, and transmission is increased by wet skin.

Molluscum appears as umbilicated pearly or skin-coloured papules and can affect any part of the body (Figure 44.4). Mollusca usually last around 6 months and then undergo spontaneous regression, but can last up to 2 years. Diagnosis is usually clinical and no treatment is required, although curette, cautery or cryosurgery can be used.

▶ Diagnoses not to be missed

Erythroderma (generalised exfoliative dermatitis)

This is a dermatological emergency characterised by scaling erythematous dermatitis involving 90% or more of the skin's surface (Figure 44.5). Causes can include primary dermatological diseases (e.g. psoriasis, atopic dermatitis), drugs or as the result of lymphoma, leukaemia, or staphylococcal scalded skin syndrome.

Complications include skin infection, hypoalbuminaemia (protein loss from skin and gut), high-output cardiac failure and impaired thermoregulation. Urgent referral to a dermatologist is necessary if this is suspected.

Stevens–Johnson syndrome

This is an immune-complex-mediated hypersensitivity complex (Figure 44.6). It ranges from mild skin and mucous membrane lesions to a severe, sometimes fatal systemic disorder. It typically involves the skin and the mucous membranes. There may be significant involvement of mouth, nose, eye, vagina, urethra, gastrointestinal tract and lower respiratory tract mucous membranes.

Meningococcal septicaemia

Meningococcal disease can occur at any age, but babies and children less than 5 years of age are most at risk. The hallmark symptoms of meningococcal septicaemia are fever and rash. Meningococcemic rash is non-blanching, develops rapidly and usually appears on the armpits, groin and ankles, and does not fade under pressure (see Figure 44.7). It is important that treatment be started as soon as possible if meningococcal disease is suspected.

Index

Page numbers in *italics* denote figures, those in **bold** denote tables.